Seduction club: Sex for free

in 7 hours

Master the art
of seduction
and make any
woman desire
you in 7 hours
or less

Book Description

Do you want to know how to seduce a woman in seven hours or less? In this book, I am going to show you exactly what to do to achieve this goal and enjoy intimate moments of pleasure, without wasting your time. There are carefully laid-out steps that you should follow from the way you approach a woman to what you tell her and how you follow up after your acquaintance, so that you maximize your odds of success and ultimately live up to the challenge.

Women are not that hard to get, as long as you push the right buttons and know how to behave. Instead of leaving everything to chance, prepare your strategy. Study the patterns of women's behavior and interpret the signs that show you whether or not she is into you. Do not rely on wishful thinking and do not stay idle. Take matters into your own hands and you will soon notice a significant change in your life. It is all about your mentality. Build up your self-confidence and know your strengths and weaknesses. And above all, set realistic targets that you can obtain, once you put your mind into them.

This book introduces you to the world of women, revealing their secrets and unmasking their guards. Truth is out there and you can make the most out of flirting, when you know where to look. Aren't you intrigued? Then what are you waiting for? Keep reading and change your life forever. You are most welcome!

Table of Contents

Table of Contents

Introduction

Are you tired of trying to find the right moves and the proper things to say to a woman? Do you feel like you do not project the image of an exciting guy that is worth getting to know? Well, navigating the dating scene can be tough, especially if you do not believe in yourself. Listen, it takes time to build up your confidence and eventually find the companionship you are seeking. But in the end, those who dare are the ones that reap the benefits of their bravery. Those who choose to act are far more likely to succeed in their goals, than those that remain idle and watch life pass them by.

So when it comes to women, what do you choose to be? Would you rather stay in the background and watch other men enchanting the most beautiful women out there? Or are you ready to fight and show the world what you are made of? If it is the latter, then I am very happy that you have selected my book to find the guidance that you need. I will do my best to present all the steps in getting acquainted, arranging your first date and making sure that you score. And all that in seven hours – tops. Does that sound too good to be true? Well, bear with me and you will see how you can accomplish this milestone easily and without drawing on pure luck. Luck has nothing to do with your hard work and efforts.

As you will get to see, this book has got everything it takes to master the art of seduction. By following the instructions and tips that I lay out in detail, you will be able to talk to any woman you like. Even if you get goosebumps at first, you will get the chance to improve your conversational skills and overcome that fear of rejection that is holding you back from showing the world what you are made of. Keep in mind that there is pain, whenever there is gain. Take on the challenge and you will see you are going to reach your end goal much sooner than anticipated.

Read through each chapter and keep notes, as they will come in handy later. It doesn't matter if you are a younger or an older guy; it doesn't matter how much money you make or what car you drive; it all boils down to your self-confidence and the pedestal you must put yourself on. You first need to appreciate the person in front of your mirror, before getting others to understand your true value. Focus on how awesome you are and work on boosting your ego. Not in a negative way, but in a healthy manner that allows you to comprehend that you are unique and that any woman would be happy to know you better...let alone sleep with you!

Time Is Money

Life can be hectic at times. You wake up early in the morning and by noon you feel like you have had enough. By night time, you are exhausted and drained of all your energy. There are too many things to do that drive you crazy. In this frenzy, you cannot expect to add more stress and anxiety into the mix. Time is money, as I am sure that you have heard again and again. This is true, since time is much too precious to waste on things that do not make a difference in the end. Why wait for a miracle to happen, when you can take matters into your own two hands and fore-shadow the end result? Yes, you have that power!

You may think that seven hours is not adequate time to see if a woman is truly into you. But I am not talking about realizing if she is the right one to marry or even carry on a steady relation-ship with. I am just letting you know if you have any chances with that woman. Otherwise, why bother? You will have plenty of other opportunities ahead, without getting fixated on a lost cause. This might sound materialistic at first, but the truth is that it points out just how valuable time is. You should not waste your days, trying to change a woman's mind and to convince her to give you a chance. No way, this is not happening. Instead, she should be coming towards you and asking to find out more about who you are. This is the correct mentality that you need to master, for the optimal outcome when it comes to sex and fe-male seduction. By the time we're done, you will have the skills to seduce a woman in seven hours – whether that is over one long date or several shorter ones.

This is a matter of self-preservation. You cannot persevere, unless you have the faintest chance of success. Think of it as a mind game. If she does not respond to your calling, then you should readjust your radar and flirt with a woman that appreciates your company. There is nothing wrong with that. Rejection should not be regarded as something disheartening. On the contrary, it should be welcome as an opportunity to grow and perfect your skills, although not at the expense of your well-being. Think of what could have gone better and modify your patterns accord-ingly next time. Improve your skills, gain invaluable experience and minimize your losses. This can only happen if you do not waste your time flirting with a woman that is not available.

Set out on this once-in-a-lifetime journey of enhancing your self worth and believing in yourself. This is a game changer, to say the least. It is going to help you broaden your horizons and enable you to see things from a different perspective. No matter if you have had plenty of steady relationships or casual sex so far, you may have never addressed the elephant in the room. You have never actually questioned the way you look at yourself and therefore you have not had the opportunity to address any issues with your self-esteem. But believing in you is the number one thing you ought to do, so as to increase your odds of success in seducing women, without wasting endless hours steeped in insecurity and doubt.

A Mind Blowing Journey Has Started

I know that many of you do not believe in yourselves. The journey to self-worth and acknowledgement is not an easy one to make. However, you cannot expect to improve your life without first realizing your value as a person. If you think that there are things that you should do differently, then what is stopping you from changing them? Life is not meant to be still and static.
No, it is meant to flow constantly in various directions that keep surprising you. This is the quintessence of life, being unpredictable and full of new things, new aspects and new opportunities. Seize every moment, right?
No one is claiming that they can predict life 100 percent of the time and see what is coming without any room for error. What I am trying to teach you here in this book is how to interpret the signs and how to dig deeper into the true meaning of female behavioral patterns. Furthermore, I am trying to show you how you can optimize your flirting skills and make a great impression on the woman you want to seduce. It is all about this first impression, which is either going to pave the way for your future trek towards happiness – even for a brief encounter – or set you on the path towards failure.
Through self-discovery, you get to see things in a new way. It is a sort of enlightenment, if you ask me. Obviously, you need to work with yourself and this alone takes time and effort. In fact, it is a

constant struggle towards self-improvement. Personal relationships are a reflection of the way you feel about yourself. The less you know about who you really are and what you are made of, the less you can hope to cultivate healthy personal relationships. And I do not just mean sexual relationships (although this is where we focus here), but also every other type of interaction with people. And unless you believe in your value, don't take it for granted that others will. It is a vicious cycle you need to escape. However, the more you learn about yourself and your inner power, the more you get to appreciate that. And once that vicious cycle ends and you find the tunnel of self-awareness in the distance, you will see how to change your life and establish relationships according to your own terms. Surely you know how precious it is to feel good about yourself. It has been inscribed in every throw pillow and it is a part of the text of any motivational speech ever delivered. But this does not do it justice, either. Because knowing yourself is the alpha and omega of happiness. You cannot be happy or exude joy to others, if you are not happy deep inside. And hopefully this book drives you towards discovering that inner happiness and bringing it to the surface.

This journey that has already begun has been designed to open your eyes to whole new horizons and allow you to see things in a different perspective. Rather than relying purely on randomness and fortune, you should concentrate on your own powers and build a solid strategy that works every single time. So keep reading and enjoy the guidelines, along with the examples and case studies that I am laying out for you to see!

Chapter 1
Know Yourself

Every person is unique and it is vital that you understand that. We do not all love basketball or fishing, nor do we all dress the same way. Some may choose casual T-shirts and jeans, while others prefer more formal outfits, wearing shirts, vests and ties. There are endless differences among people, in the way they eat and drink, the way they choose to spend their free time and, of course, differences in their personal preferences. Some want a 4x4 vehicle and others choose sports cars or even SUVs. I could go on and on about each person's unique character and personality, but you get the idea. We are all different entities in the world.

In a universe where uniformity is celebrated and everybody strives to fit in, I know that it can be hard to acknowledge what you are made of. But as you grow older and more mature, you ought to pursue the discovery of your true self without any hidden agenda. You owe it to yourself to stay true. Embrace your uniqueness, but only after you have fully comprehended who you really are. Identify your strengths and weaknesses and find out what you really love or hate. See the principles that you have always lived by, evaluate them and realize if your priorities need any reassessment.

Only after having found yourself, can you build the confidence it takes to succeed in your goals. And these goals are not limited

to charming women and luring them to have sex with you
in seven hours or less. They vary greatly, covering both your
personal and professional life. A man who knows who he is can
conquer the world. This is the mentality you are after, isn't it?
So, in order to be successful in seducing a woman, you first need
to be confident enough that you understand that a woman
is not doing you any favors by agreeing to go out with you.
It is that special uniqueness, the sum of all your traits and features, the smallest details that make a huge difference and
comprise your amazing self. You cannot expect everyone to
look the same, feel the same or be the same. Instead, you must
comprehend that being unique is a blessing and not something
to shy away from. But first things first. Who are you, in your very
essence?

Who are you, really? Have you ever wondered who you truly are
and, most importantly, who you want to be? These are fundamental questions that you should have answered, prior to setting
out on your journey to seduce a woman's heart. Women couldn't
care less for men that are indecisive, insecure and lacking
self-esteem. Instead, believing in yourself and your self-worth
is the absolute aphrodisiac for them. They are attracted by the
alpha male and this is not just a stereotype. Alpha males are
quite dominant and know what they are after. They do not rely
on the judgment of other people's choices, as they are clearly
trying to shape their own destiny.

Dominance over your life is essential. You should take charge of
things happening in your life and influence others, rather than
be influenced by them. Why follow the trends when you can set
your own trends over time and appear as a pioneer? I know that
it may sound intimidating, but think about the ultimate sense
of independence that you would get to feel when you are freed
from the chains that you have put yourself into. It feels like a revelation – a revelation that is inevitably transformed into a yearning
to introduce women to the man that they deserve...you!
Clearly, this is something that you have to work on full speed.
I mean, figuring out who you are is fundamental in a number

of different scenarios. But here we are talking about women and their impact on you. Not all men will fight over the same type of women, this makes sense. Therefore, you must first narrow down your spectrum and see which of these women make your mind blow. In a nutshell, you really need to identify your type of woman.

Identify Your Type of Women

When it comes to women, options are equally chaotic to all other choices you will be expected to make in your life. Each man needs to have a clear picture in his mind as to what he wants. You do not need to exclude blondes or brunettes altogether. In fact, it is healthy to keep an open mind about these options, in terms of how each woman looks. Of course, you may have a soft spot for freckles or curvy bodies, short hair or women wearing glasses. It is perfectly OK to embrace these preferences of yours, since they will motivate you to try even harder to achieve your end goal.

There are men that do not dare to flirt with a woman, if they feel that she is out of their league. Are you one of those folks? If so, then get a grip! Women couldn't care less about your looks. Or to be more accurate, it is not their top priority to find somebody that looks like he just got out of a photo shoot for the cover of a magazine. Sure, a six-pack has never hurt a man in getting laid. Yet, this is not why he gets lucky in the first place. There are much more crucial elements in the mix that a woman seeks in a man, which means that you should not limit your prey, because you think that they belong to men who are more handsome than you. Chances are that you will see them walking hand in hand with a man that is not as good looking as you.

So back to the ladies. Have you concluded as to who you prefer? Obviously, these are just preferences and they do not restrict you from flirting with others. But it is very helpful to understand what your type is, so as to minimize your target audience and focus on the women that you like. Too many options can confuse you, even if you do not realize that. Plus, there are some truly basic things to consider about a woman's looks that either excite or turn you off. For instance, some men appreciate a woman with big breasts and others admire long legs. There is nothing wrong with either of these choices, but they do form an excluding trend. You can either like a girl that is taller than you or not. In general, men tend to repeat those choices of theirs in their life. So what is your type of woman?

Of course, everyone has his own preferences in terms of what types of women do you like, such as a domestic goddess, a self-sufficient career woman or a sports-loving tom girl. Maybe you see yourself with a hybrid of these women or another type. We all have our comfort zones in dress, in hobbies, in work and, of course, in relationships. So let's not aim to hook you up with a librarian in a fully buttoned blouse who will hardly pay attention to a man who feels more relaxed in loose shorts and comfy slippers. The right women are out there, waiting for you!

It is not just about the looks, though. Every woman takes pride in her individual personality, but you could say that there are categories of women you may like or choose to steer clear of. For instance, some men particularly love sweet-talking women who are sensitive and caring. On the other hand, there are women that appear to be especially dynamic and powerful so they catch the attention of other men. In a similar pattern, you can evaluate various categories and see if you find them appealing or if you feel turned off by them. In the process, you may be surprised about the things that you characterize as attractive. And looking back on your previous choices, you will most probably notice a pattern unveiling itself in front of you.

Well, the ball is in your hands now. What is it that you love about women? And on the other hand, what is it that totally puts you off? You need to realize if you enjoy being with a bossy woman or with a woman that does not want to have the upper hand in a relationship. There is no shame in either of these cases, obviously. But comprehending your type of woman brings you a little closer to your target. Why fool around with a housewife, when clearly you are not meant to be together? Even if at first you like her, you are only delaying the inevitable!

Seduction Lies in the Details

OK, you have narrowed down your options as to which woman makes your heart run wild. This is a good first step, since it allows you to separate the wheat from the chaff and only focus on the type of woman that you truly enjoy having by your side. Be it an acquaintance for one night or for the rest of your life (just saying), you should not settle for someone that does not appeal to you. And now, it is time to concentrate on the seduction. How do you expect to seduce a woman, unless you believe in your own value? So before going ahead with the step by step guide on how to make any woman fall for you in less than seven hours, let's talk about you.

Are you happy with the way you look, the way you talk and the way you walk? If you aren't, then you should do something about it. A man like you should ooze self-esteem and certainty. These are the elements that you need to work on, because they are fundamental in your effort to win a woman's heart. Luckily, you can boost your confidence and build trust in you, but it takes time and it requires full dedication. No self-doubting here, man. This will put you in an inferior position, trying to convince a woman about something that you do not actually believe in.

As the title suggests, seduction lies in the details. So make sure that you pay attention to those little touches. It doesn't have to be a true transformation of your looks, since this is not important. But it is essential that you look your best. This means that from now on you cannot expect to leave your beard untrimmed, your hair uncombed and your skin unnourished. Come on, you should be celebrating. Now is the time for you to shine and indulge in some long-anticipated care. Think of it as promotion of goods. How can you sell a product, if it appears to be all dirty and unkempt?

Seduction club

Apart from a makeover of your beauty care routine, you should also show close attention to what you are wearing. This is your identity, a reflection of who you are and what matters to you. Again, you do not need to go overboard. Nevertheless, it would be great if your clothes and accessories told a story for you. This tale will fascinate women and intrigue them to get to know you better. It is not necessary to spend a small fortune to elevate your style, so why don't you? Go shopping and see what truly suits you, rather than what you may have tricked yourself into liking. For instance, you can get away with stamped T-shirts if you are a teen. But seriously? If you want to convey the message that you are a man worth exploring, then why on Earth would you buy a T-shirt that contradicts everything you are trying hard to exude? Instead, introduce collared shirts to your wardrobe, if you are not a fan of them already. They look classy and they vary greatly, from casual to formal and everything in between. A nice pair of jeans is quite versatile, if you avoid patches and holes. Next, do not under-estimate the power of great shoes. They show that you pay atten-tion to details, so feel free to invest some money and get shoes that radiate sophistication. Add a few accessories like a branded watch to make a huge difference in the end result.
It goes without even saying that you should be yourself.
Still, with some careful moves you will improve your looks and maintain that charming personality of yours at the same time. If you want to seduce a woman, you need to come across as a confident man, who is bold and daring. Your stylistic options highlight your taste and mentality to an extent. So with just a few twists here and there, you can rest assured that the first stages of seduction go as planned. It is so worth it, plus you will feel extra fine wearing clothes that enhance your masculinity and your awesomeness.

Chapter 2
Where to Meet

Now that you have cleared the air as to what type of woman makes your heart go wild, we move forward with the next step. I imagine that you have been out to innumerable dates, some of which have ended up in absolute disaster! Although a first date seems straightforward, it can indeed make or break your relationship right from the outset. Be it a one-night stand, a casual flirt or the beginning of a wonderful companionship, it all starts here. Just the thought of sharing the spicy details of this rendezvous with your kids or grandkids (yeah, I know I have gone too far!) raises expectations. Can you keep up? I am sure you can!

So what makes a date epic and what turns it into an epic fail? Well, the first thing that you need to remember is to keep things simple. In fact, there is no room for pretentious behavior during the first date. On the contrary, play it cool. Rather than trying to find sophisticated restaurants where you can dine under the stars or opera performances that neither of you truly appreciate, get your feet back on the ground. Be realistic and think of what you enjoy in a night out. Unless the answer involves mud wrestling or loud

You should aim for creativity. Put your very own personal touch in the date. It does not have to be something fancy, rather than a minor detail that sets this date apart from all the others. Are you intrigued? Now, spend a moment in her shoes and think how she will feel, knowing that you went the extra mile to prepare something special for her. A picnic might sound weird to you, but the open air and the proximity to nature drive women wild. Or better yet, a special surprise that you prepare for her eyes only can be your secret and earn you some points. She does not need to know that you have done the exact same thing for a dozen other women!

However, the question remains. Where should you meet for the first time? Which is the ideal place for a first date and why? Even though your unique self may beg to differ, there are some places that truly hit the spot and maximize your odds to seduce the woman you desire. Avoid the minefields and select one of these options, getting closer to your trophy. As you will see, there are quite a few options for you to choose from. These options will help you keep things smooth and fine throughout the date. And above all, they will allow you to communicate and discover many things about each other. So which are those places and why should you opt for one of them?

Perfect Places to Meet & Those Better to Avoid

One of the safest choices is for you to meet at a bar.
There is nothing fancy about it, but special details can go a long way. First of all, you can go to a pub that you know very well. This means that you control the environment 100 percent and you are very likely to impress her with free shots! More than that, you have a great topic to talk about, such as the remarkable history of this hidden gem or some things that only "few" people know. It will add a sense of mystery and adventure to the date, for sure. Of course, after a few drinks, you can either part ways or suggest going to your place. But beware! When meeting at a bar, you always risk drinking too much. Obviously you can hold your liquor, but the lady might fall off the wagon, especially if she is

feeling nervous or she is having too much of a good time. Perhaps a walking date is not the first one on your list. However, you should give it a try. Find a place worth discovering on foot and enjoy a stroll together. You can grab a cup of coffee or even a cocktail for the road, accompanied with salty or sweet snacks. The best thing is that walking helps you relax and the fresh air makes you feel alive. Depending on the time of year, you can admire the sunset colors in the sky or a starlit night or get sun-kissed while having a "brunch to go." When you get tired, there are always benches where you can sit down and continue your breezy talk. Nevertheless, you should make sure that the woman knows where you are going. Do not attempt to surprise her, because it is likely that she will be wearing high heels or an outfit that does not encourage even the mildest workout.

A mall is another place to meet. Although every cell in your body is telling you to ignore that, just hear me out. First off, there are tons of things to do there. You can go shopping and make funny comments while trying out scarves, hats or accessories. The foodcourt and specialty shops feature plenty of food and drink options. You can chat and bond over a cup of coffee, share a piece of decadent chocolate cake or enjoy dinner and cocktails in a friendly and familiar atmosphere. There are few surprises there, which is good to help with the stress that you may experience prior to your rendezvous. On the other hand, some people think that branded chain restaurants and cafes lack personality and therefore they should be avoided on a first (second, third, you get the gist) date.

Meeting at a party is always a good option, since the vibe is already positive and you will both have something in common. A party organized at a college event, an office get-together or a reunion are all special events to be celebrated with colleagues and peers. These are some of the reasons why parties are so popular. So if this is the case and you notice a beautiful girl standing alone in the distance, you would be a mad man not to go over to her. "Hi, how do you know Jake?" is a decent opening line. "This party is pretty entertaining, wouldn't you say so?" or

Seduction club

"I see that you are not drinking. How else do you expect to tolerate this music?" are also great conversation starters, with a personal twist. Then, depending on her answer, you can go ahead with more details. And be sure not to say anything sarcastic or diminishing for somebody at the party. After all, you don't really know who she is here with!

Last but not least, there is a place that I bet you have not thought of. Are you ready? Well, it is your home and hers. At the same time. Or your office and her backyard, the beach or an Internet cafe. Can you guess where I am going with this? In this era that is overwhelmed by technology, it is an option that you make great use of such technological advancements and enjoy a tech-friendly first date remotely. You can use Skype or Facebook Messenger, Viber or WhatsApp or basically any app or social media platform appeals to you the most. In this way, you can get to know each other while talking and exchanging opinions, without experiencing the awkwardness of physical contact. After all, you will be in an environment that is familiar to you, so you will not feel threatened or cause her to feel uneasy. Obviously, this type of date is most suitable for younger age groups. And under no circumstances can it be compared to the pleasure you get from meeting somebody face to face. But it can work, especially if you love technology and getting online!

Now that you know where to take that special lady out on a first date, why don't we also point out where not to go? Better safe than sorry, right? Well, one of the worst places to go would definitely be the cinema. Do I need to state the obvious? There are many bad things about it. First, you will not get the chance to talk and connect with each other. Sure, you can share the popcorn, but that's about it! How can you seduce a woman, when you are sitting next to her, avoiding even the slightest eye contact? Plus, you can never know if she appreciates the same movies as you (which, let's face it, almost never happens). If you hit it off and get to be a couple, then movie nights take on a whole new meaning and you will love them. For now, put them aside.

A night at home might sound idyllic. Nevertheless, it is the absolute no-no when it comes to first dates. You will need to make sure that everything is spotlessly clean, without any trace of female presence and with the right balance between your masculine side and her more sophisticated aesthetics. Furthermore, you will most likely have to cook for her and create the perfect ambiance, when both of you are somewhat nervous and the stakes are too high. Let's not forget that your bedroom is just around the corner - literally! Even though you would think this is an advantage, it can turn into disaster as soon as you make the first move.

I don't know why I feel the need to say this, but you should NEVER bring a girl to your parents' house on your first date. Well, there are some men that feel the internal urge to get approval from their parents. If you are one of those men, then you surely need some serious changes in the way you think. Parents are great – I love mine – but it is good to set up some clearly defined boundaries. You should not subject your lovely lady to a date where you get to know each other, under the prying eyes of her "future in-laws." Moreover, you will be sending the wrong message to your folks too and this is not fair. So stay away from your parents' house. You can go there to ask for food, money, laundry or to check up on them. However, this is hardly the place to go out on a romantic night.

Finally, you had better steer clear of anything too fancy. This includes a wide range of places, but it is best to avoid them all! Extraordinary ethnic cuisine, amusement parks with roller coasters (unless you are teens) and karaoke, ice skating or even your cousin's wedding are all out of the question. Choose something less overwhelming and go with the flow in this case. Hopefully, by the end of your date you will have realized whether or not this lady likes that kind of extravagant stuff. Again, you should stop thinking about how to impress her for all the wrong reasons and focus on what is important. The quintessence of a successful first date is establishing communication and getting to know each other in a pleasant ambiance.

Online Dating: Does It Work?

Nowadays, technology has dominated our lives and there is no turning back. Why would it be, after all? You can find everything online – shop and search for all sorts of information, book tickets and buy memorabilia. The Internet is powerful and it has in fact revolutionized the way we communicate with each other. And along with all the benefits that society gets from the Internet, online dating holds a special place. There are many people that find it better to flirt online and avoid that physical presence of a date face to face. But is it really a thing? Can you base your hopes of seducing a woman to a computer, a smartphone or a tablet? The Internet comes with its pros and cons and online dating is no different. If you are feeling insecure about the way you look or if you are having trouble talking to a woman, especially a woman that you like, then online dating can come to the rescue. In this way, you can overcome your fears and hesitations. Indeed, the physical barrier of a technological wonder in the form of an electronic gadget makes the whole experience less nerve wracking. Furthermore, through the Internet you can choose what to say and when to say it. You control the environment and the timing. Actually, you are pretty much in control of everything, compared to what can happen out in public. Isn't that great?

Furthermore, in online dating you can specify exactly what it is that you are searching for at the moment. There are men and women that are only looking for casual sex. They are in pursuit of sexual pleasure, with no strings attached. In that case, you know what to anticipate. When a woman is in the mood for sex, her expectations in the field of seduction are pretty low. This means that you do not have to spend time thinking about what to say and how to react to her signals. You both know what is about to happen, don't you? So why pretend it is something entirely different? If you are looking for temporary satisfaction, then you can check online dating out and look for like-minded women. In fact, you can narrow down your search as per age group, marital status or even location.

Every coin has two sides and therefore you should consider the drawbacks of online dating, prior to deciding if you should give it a chance. First of all, the lack of a personal touch can be disastrous. In this book, I have told you over and over again that you must highlight your awesomeness and unique personality. But how can you do that over the net? It can be far too difficult. More than that, you cannot impress her through your posture, your clothes and the way you walk and talk. Why wear that signature cologne, when there is no way for her to smell it? How can you interpret her body language and receive all these signals that she is sending you, when the only thing that you can exchange online is emojis?

Nonetheless, a deeper thing lies beneath the surface and prevents me from recommending online dating as the best practice. Even though it can help you communicate and schedule a date with a woman, a real problem persists. If you are not confident enough to support your direct approach to a woman face to face, then how can you expect to seduce her in seven hours or less? How can you expect to overcome those fears that have been creeping up on you all these years, holding you back from claiming hot dates filled with sex? Unless you assess the situation and identify the problem, you will not be able to fix it. Online dating is simply a substitute for what you are after. Think about what matters to you the most. Are you interested in taking the shortcut, without evidently mending what is broken? Or are you willing to push yourself more, creating solid foundations for your future self? There is no right or wrong here, but you need to remain true to your mission.

If you decide to stick to online dating, you might want to know how to beat competition and increase the chances of your desired woman talking to you. It is true that there are many many other men out there, in search of the very same thing. They are looking for a woman to hook up with and they are very straightforward about it. So you need to figure out how to come across as special and worth talking to online. How can you do that? The Internet can be cruel and you only get one chance to do it right, when approaching her and starting a conversation. It is common for men to use the very same punchlines with all the women that they talk to. In this way, they minimize the time and mental effort that they need to approach a woman. Plus, who can think of a different line to send to 100 different ladies? It is nearly impossible, unless you are a writer or you have plenty of time to kill. So, since we have rejected that option, we can move forward with what you should actually use to catch her attention online.

First of all, you should avoid generic comments like "You look so beautiful!" or "How come you are here online? Men should be lining up to meet you!" at all costs. You do not want to appear as trying to make up for a lack of self-esteem. After all, there is nothing wrong with online dating and therefore you should not be ashamed or belittle yourself by acknowledging that you are searching for an online hookup. In a similar pattern, she should not be judged for being here at the same place, looking for the same thing. No matter if she is super hot or just cute, she might really like online dating or this could be the perfect timing for you both.

One great rule of thumb would be to keep it simple and classy, with a touch of humor and creativeness but still without anything too much. Does that even make sense? You can start a conversation by complimenting her in an indirect manner. If you are wondering how to do this, here are some examples that you can use. You can tell her that she is very cute and that her smile just made you smile, too. Or you can compliment her on the profile photo that she has uploaded, telling her that it brings out her artistic side. Of course, there is also the option of using humor as your secret weapon. "Girl, I will get in so much trouble when I introduce you to my mum!" or "Ok, you've got me. I will go out with you!" can earn you some points for creativity, which is not a bad thing to do!

Chapter 3
Reading Women

For most men, women are a total mystery. They appear to be complex human beings, meant to puzzle men with their behavior and leaving them at a loss. Their mind works in mysterious ways, while they are emotional creatures who tend to overthink even the most trivial of things. Even though the stereotypes are not always right, in this case they can speak louder than words. There are miles separating men and women, which is why most of us are left wondering what we should have done differently. But is it really so hard?

It goes without even saying that women are emotional. They rely a great deal on their instincts and sometimes they act on an impulse, driven by what their heart dictates. Sure, there is also logic and in most cases it comes through friendly advice, since women tend to share details about their personal life and seek help from their trusted besties. And sometimes it would appear that women act in an irrational manner. But this is only if you just scratch the surface and do not dig deeper. Once you do, you will realize that their behavior is most likely justifiable. OK, I know, I know there are always exceptions to this rule!

When it comes to relationships, things can be less awkward when you are aware of what to expect. Fully comprehending the psychology of a woman will allow you to be a step ahead and anticipate what is coming. Isn't that wonderful? Rather than fear for the worst--case scenario, you should study how women react, how they behave and what they want. You don't have to be Mel Gibson (well, it wouldn't hurt either!) to get inside a woman's mind. It is all there, waiting for you to interpret. A woman reveals her secrets when she is around you. She sends messages, subtle yet distinctive ones, guiding you to the right moves.

Having sex is a very important milestone for men and women alike. Yet, women seem to have more issues to deal with when it comes to sex with a stranger than men. They put too much pressure on themselves, in pursuit of the perfect balance between ethics and desire. On the one hand, they think that first date sex can ruin their reputation or at least send out the wrong message about their values and morality; on the other hand, though, they hate to be characterized as a puritan or a person that refuses to indulge in something clearly fun and pleasurable.

So all you have to do is learn how to read between the lines, understand what these signs are and ultimately "read women." You will be able to identify the signals that they are sending to you and act as per what they actually want. This skill will turn out to be extra handy, since you will know when to step up your game and when to hold back for a while. Yes, it won't happen overnight; but it will unfold gradually, offering you a unique opportunity to get closer and really evaluate the situation. "Is she into me?" Why ask this question again and again, when you can open up your eyes and see for yourself?

Is She Into You?

Obviously, you are not a mind reader! However, there are some patterns in her behavior that will unveil the mystery of attraction to you. So imagine that you are in a bar, enjoying a drink with your friends. Your eyes are wandering, until you spot that lovely lady looking at you. This can be random. But wait! What happened when you stared back at her? Did she get embarrassed, startled or even blush? And most importantly, did she continue looking at you? Maybe even smiled or nodded? These are all signs that a woman is interested in you.

So what are you waiting for? Follow up on what she has started, smiling or even raising your glass for a "remote toast." If she looks the other way, then it is a hard pass. If not, then this can be the beginning of an acquaintance. Build up your courage and self-esteem, getting over there to introduce yourself. Obviously, this can play out in a million different ways and not all of them are great. But instead of doubting yourself, pick up that discreet body language and make your move.

When you do approach her, again read the signs. Check if she is nervous and use an ice-breaker to get that discussion flowing. You do not need to worry about being creative and imaginative. Hopefully, you will have all the time in the world to do that. Now keep things simple. Chat and if you see her as a great fit, then ask for her number. Then, you can plan when to text or call, what to say and how to proceed. After your question, observe her reactions. Is she playing it cool or is she hesitant to give you the number? Is she timid, or is she thinking of a nice way to refuse? Body language is there, just know where to look!

Case study: There is a woman that touches her hair and tosses her curls back, revealing her neckline and cheeks. She slightly closes her eyelids, while still keeping contact with your eyes. When you talk, she leans her head on one side and bites or licks her lips. She touches you for a moment and smiles. And above all, she laughs! These are all signs that a woman likes you and wants intimacy. In fact, she is using nature to her advantage, even if she doesn't even realize that. Hair and neck are filled with pheromones, which she drives towards you. Closing her eyes and turning attention to her lips will lead you subconsciously to the act of human pleasure. Aren't these hints enough for you?

Some women are more accustomed to using their body language and play out these signs more intensely, whereas others are less confident and do not even know what their body is telling you. In general, people tend to allow closer contact with those that appeal to them. So if she lets you into her personal space, this is a very encouraging step. Go slowly, though. Do not plunge right in, or else you risk scaring her off. Instead, go with the flow and when you spot something sketchy on her facial expressions or if you see that she is taking a step back, follow her lead and relax. Have you ever been fishing? Then you know the feeling. There are many signs that you should observe in a woman, when she is talking to you or even before approaching her. A woman that is well aware of her sexual nature will be open to show you what she wants. Her clothes will most likely point it out, too. You may notice that she has unbuttoned the two first buttons of her shirt. Perhaps she has slightly opened her legs, motivating you to look just for a second or two, until she closes them again. Wetting her lips is another indication that she is in the mood for sex. And another thing; observe how she is holding the straw or how her fingers are touching the glass of her drink. This might give you an idea as to where she is headed.

If I had to give you just one piece of advice, this would be to stop listening with your ears to what a woman wants. It is just like trusting her when she is telling you that she doesn't want anything for her birthday. Well, as soon as she spells this out, you know it is a lie, right? Well, it is the same here. Her body language is shouting at you, if you only learn how to listen. You need to practice before perfecting your skills. And beware of distracting yourself too much with her body language, which may be misinterpreted as lack of interest. A man that does not pay attention to what she says is not a man to treasure, right? So tread lightly and preserve the balance between understanding what she wants non-verbally and still communicating with her verbally.

No-No Signs

You have got closer to her and you have employed all your charms, so that she falls for it and you reap the benefits of your seduction skills. But instead, you feel like you are talking to a wall of concrete. She does not seem to share the same enthusiasm as you, when you talk. In fact, she seems uninspired to continue the conversation. No matter what you say, her reactions are quite dull and repetitive. Her replies are short and firm, there is no chemistry between you and clearly it is far from "love at first sight." But you really fancy her. What do you do?

This is not a happy topic to discuss, but it is essential for you to avoid investing more time and energy into a lost cause. When a woman is not interested, it is best that you move on. You can always try to reverse the situation, building lust and desire. Still, the odds are not in your favor and you should not be offended by that. There are a lot more fish in the sea, for sure! You remember the topic of this book, don't you? Time is ticking and you should put that into the equation, before you decide what to do with this woman. But how can you be sure that she is not into you, rather than playing hard to get? Luckily, her body language will tell you all about it from day one.

Basically, check out where she keeps her hands and what she does with them. Does she keep them folded in front of her chest or maybe she is connecting the ends of her fingers at a crazy speed? Then this is an indication that she preserves her distance from you. She wants to withhold her personal space and makes sure that you do not intrude. Or maybe she is using the phone a lot, and I mean a lot! Even while you are talking, she is checking her inbox or getting selfies for her Instagram. She is scrolling down to read all about her friends' activities, laughing at the pictures and commenting on posts. She is clearly searching for a distraction. The same goes for touching her hair and searching for split ends (yes, many women do that, but not during a potentially romantic situation). And don't get me started on keeping her hands in her pockets.

Facial expressions can be cruel, but they give you more than a hint as to whether or not you have a chance. If you see a woman frowning or making that famous "duck face" without trying to kiss you, then she is bothered by your presence or by what you are saying. And this often comes hand in hand with rolling eyes, along with general strict face and posture. Her eyebrows are another indication as to whether or not she is attracted to you. Raising one eyebrow is definitely a warning sign, whereas slightly raising both and lowering her eyelids are the exact opposite. Moreover, if you notice that she sighs a lot, yawns or huffs and puffs, well it is a no-brainer that this is not a woman for you. So do not prolong the inevitable and end your interaction, before it turns into a complete nightmare for your ego (Lovz, 2019).

One more thing that you should keep in mind is that some women enjoy friendzoning men, at least at the beginning of their acquaintance. Well, personally I do not like that and so I move on, without ever looking back. My intentions are clear from the start, hence there is no room for mixed signals. However, you can be fine with that. It is true that a friendship can grow into something much more than that and it takes time. Given that, when you are on a strict time frame, you ought to be crystal clear as to the signals you both receive and send out. How can you compromise with being her friend, when evidently the first thing that you thought of when looking at her was to tear her clothes apart and find out how her skin tastes? Again, stay focused on your goal. You need to make her yours in seven hours tops. When she is friendzoning you, this can never happen. It is up to you to call it off or simply allow her to be your friend, but do not keep your hopes up.

All these signs tell you that a woman is not interested in talking to you or, more precisely, she is not interested in becoming your sex partner. Fair enough. No harm done. You need to realize that this is not the end of the world, nor should it be a blow to your bruised ego. She doesn't know you, maybe she is already in a relationship or she is trying to recover after a bad breakup. Or she wants to dedicate her time to school or work, putting flirt aside for a while. There are many different things that can be going on, most of which have absolutely NOTHING to do with you. So instead of taking it personally and trying hard to figure out why she is not receptive to your attempt to approach her, just forget about it and keep the ball rolling.

Chapter 4
What to Say after "Hello"

Imagine that you have found the woman you want to ask out
and you want to approach her. You build up your courage,
like we talked about earlier, and you are getting closer and closer.
It makes sense that your heart starts pounding faster, your heart
rate has gone through the roof. Or at least, you don't feel comfortable about the situation - but that's life! Now what? How do you
play this out after saying "Hello"? Do you have a routine or a list
of things to say or do you improvise and hope for the best? If it is
the former, you had better reassess those lines. If it is the latter,
then you should remind yourself that practice makes perfect!
The way you approach the woman is definitely important.
By no means should you come off as arrogant or aggressive.
Nobody appreciates such an attitude. On the other hand, you
should not appear as too shy or lacking confidence. You are trying to "promote" yourself in a way, so you must master the skills
of a salesman. Still, one rule of thumb is to always keep it simple.
Organizing your thoughts and having some topics to discuss at
hand is a great strategy. Nonetheless, making an entrance and
starting talking with sophisticated words about something you
had to Google first to gather information is not the right way
to go. In short, be sincere.
This might sound a bit uncalled for, but I feel the need to say it.
There are men that have chosen to approach a woman from

behind. Perhaps this is the way to avoid embarrassment, since she will not be looking at them and they will have the opportunity to surprise her. But this whole thing will serve as the ultimate turnoff for her. In all likelihood, she will jump from her seat and show her shock. Who sneaks up on people and blindsides them? More than that, this move is often accompanied by touching and this is certainly not the right way to establish intimacy with a woman that you like at this stage. So even if you are shy and you want to take advantage of her lack of attention, do not creep her out. Do not come to her from behind and startle her. This is not nice, man, not nice at all!

"Hello" is a cool punching line, no matter what people claim. It is a greeting, after all - how bad can it be? Everybody is familiar with such a casual word and enables you to move forward with your next lines. And this is where you can add your personal touch and get creative. Don't be tacky, though. Unless you know for sure that she is going to love what you are saying, play it safe. There are millions of lines to use, just pick one and see how she responds. This is the key to success, always adjusting your sails according to the wind and not the other way around.

Now, rather than settling for the casual talk about the weather or asking where she is from, there are some slightly different things to consider asking. Do not lose your sleep over what to ask a woman you are interested in. If she wants to talk, she will most likely do that, no matter what you tell her. However, if you want to gain bonus points to get into her heart, then you need to devote some time and energy into that. Depending on the time and place, the age group you are targeting and even the current affairs, there is an entire treasure chest filled with topics to use. Pick the most suitable ones for you and remember that this is a marathon, not a sprint!

Another thing that you had better take into consideration when picking a topic to discuss with her, is the fact that most women appreciate a connection with the person they talk to. Find some common ground and build your conversation around that. For example, if you have both gone to the same school, focus on that and ask her about her favorite teacher or tell her that you were captain of the football team and so on. In a similar pattern, you can talk about pets and laugh at how cute your dog or kitten is. Does she love animals? Does she have a pet or what was the name of her first pet? Is she a dog or a cat person? All these questions can build a good rapport between you two and cultivate that precious feeling of connection. If you do not connect to the person in front of you, then the conversation will soon be forgotten. But if you do, it is highly likely that you will remember what you have talked about for a long time.

So rather than trying to figure out what to say next, pick up the clues that she has left for you. You will notice that she has already revealed things that you can use to your advantage. See those breadcrumbs and follow them, in order to discover your special connection. This is a sure way to a woman's heart, pointing out the things that you have in common and building trust with them as your pillars. And indeed this is a great tip for you to stand out among the rest as you seduce her, through your common ground and mutual experiences.

How to Stand Out & What Next

Besides your looks, the way you are dressed and the confidence that you are oozing, you need to practice your lines. You should know by now that the best way to a woman's heart is by conversing with her. After greeting the woman you are interested in, you can go ahead and ask her about her day. This is a rather safe topic and you will be able to see if she is open to a new acquaintance or not. "How is your day so far?" is a great way to get started. Without resorting to "Awful weather today, right?," you will manage to fuel the conversation and then move forward with juicier stuff. "Tough day at the office?" or even "Do you come here often?" can work, too. Since it is the first thing you tell her, creativity is not vital. It is welcome, though.

Seduction club

Some men are afraid of saying something good to a person,
no matter what. So they end up depriving others of some great
boost in how they are feeling. If you are like that, then I would ad-
vise you to reconsider. Compliments are always amazing and you
should not be afraid to shower the people around you with them,
but only when you see fit. Obviously, not all women are open
to compliments and you must be subtle at all times. Since this
is a stranger to you, try your best not to provoke her. You can
say something like "I really like what you are wearing" or "Great
sweater!" and watch her smile light up the room. But do not
mention that she is sexy in that dress (of course she is, of course
it is her intention to be sexy), because she may even get offended. If you want, you can pay her a compliment about her hair,
because this is one of the top things women care about, when
it comes to their looks.

Work with the surroundings, so that you are in perfect alignment
with the mood she is in. For example, if she is at a cafeteria and
she has a book with her coffee mug, it would be awesome to
ask something about that. "Is this book any good?" or "I've heard
some interesting reviews about the book, what do you think?"
Chances are good that she will appreciate the fact that you love
reading books and she will start telling you all about it. I simply
hope that this is not too boring for you. In a similar pattern, you
can comment on the music and especially if you know a thing
or two about the background song at that time. "Do you know
this song?" can work its magic and enable you to talk to her.
"Have you ever been to this part of town before?" or "Are you a fan
of Greek cuisine?" or "I am planning to buy my niece a present,
would you recommend that coloring book?" are also good and
allow you to move forward with your conversation.

It would be great if you had a story planned to narrate to her,
once you have initiated communication. This can be a funny
story or an interesting situation from the past, along with spicy
details that make the narration more pleasant. You should make
sure that you keep her interest, otherwise just cut it out. But
beware of the traps here. What you and your male friends find

interesting bears no actual resemblance with what she and her female friends would find as exciting. So no jokes or stories about farting and take fishing off the table. And under no circumstances should you use the same pick-up lines that most men use. "How did you feel falling from the sky? Are you hurt?" or "Are you tired? Because you have been in my dreams all night!" make even the sweetest woman get mad.

Another point to keep in mind is interaction. You are not meant to talk on your own, so what you say had better promote a response other than yes or no. Once you have greeted each other, why don't you ask something work-related or why don't you comment on the food, etc.? Asking her opinion is always a good strategy, too. It is all about communicating. She feels important, while you get the chance to listen to her, gathering information for your next lines. This is a win-win situation! Before you know it, you will be in sync with each other and your conversation will flow effortlessly. If you are in a bar and you are looking for a line that she may not have prepared herself for, why don't you ask her this: "What does your cocktail taste like?" and see how she responds to that. She might smile, because she has played it in her mind and is basically wondering if you are going to ask her to have a sip or suggest kissing her to have a taste. Or perhaps she just answers briefly, explaining the ingredients or something. Either way, she will answer. It is worth a try, for sure!

Whatever you choose to talk about, one thing is certain; you need to come across as confident and therefore it is essential that you speak calmly, meaning every word you are saying. It will not matter what you are saying, if your voice hardly comes out due to stress. The right line is just a vessel that allows you to move further. Even the perfect line will not do you any good, unless it is in perfect alignment with the confidence that you show the world. Your clothes, your hair, your face, your hands and palms, your shoes. These are all elements adding to the overall impression you make. And do not underestimate the power of first impressions!

Seduction club

After having successfully managed to talk to the woman you like, what should you do next? How do you proceed careful-ly, as not to waste the momentum that you have built so far? Well, typically you need to take it slowly and not rush into things. In other words, do not make the first move too fast. You can ask for her number and, assuming that she is positive to that, you can wait then follow up with a call or text. If you make your move too quickly, the results might be opposite to the ones you have been hoping for.

Follow up to what you have started building and do not shy away from the challenge. You have felt that connection, haven't you? Assuming that you have indeed sensed it and you both want to proceed with a more intimate rendezvous, then do not hold it off too long. It makes perfect sense that small talk at a nightclub does not automatically guarantee that you are going to hook up with that girl. But unless you step up your game and take the lead, how can you know for sure? The next step is equally important as the first one. After having overcome your fears to approach her, you should do the same with following up on her. Of course, there is always the option of adding her on social me-dia like Facebook, Instagram or even LinkedIn. Younger genera-tions have tons of other social media, so feel free to add the ones that you feel more comfortable using. In this way, you can check her out and see how she behaves online while being a member on those platforms, what her interests are and more. After ac-cepting your invitation to connect, you can start a casual talk that ends with you asking her out. Technology has come a long way, so it would be a shame not to take advantage of such progress! Last but definitely not least, there is the chance of her asking for your phone number or adding you to her list of friends. This is a great first step, as you can imagine. But again, do not rush things. Just appreciate the gesture and contact her in due time to evaluate the situation. And then, if everything goes as planned and her interest is evident, you ask her out. She may have done that to see if you are willing to connect with her on a more per-sonal level. Perhaps she wants to check you out online and see if you are a big flirt, as well as gather information about you and your hobbies, your preferences and your surroundings. Cool, just make sure that there is nothing there that she had better not see (like flirting with a dozen other women).

Do Not Shy Away

You have made such a great first impression and you have started showing off your true self. But it is only natural that you get cold feet at some point. Does this mean that all this hard work will go down the drain? Of course not! There is no reason why you should chicken out, after having accomplished all that. You have established your contact and you are one step closer to your target. And now it is time for your next challenge in this course of events. I believe in you, since you have already sought out help in my book to improve your moves and maximize your odds of success. So what comes next?

It is essential that you focus on your social dexterities and fight off your impulse to come across as shy. Although some women like a timid man, this is not a great indication that this man is going to be exceptional in bed. And since this ranks high on your list (as it does on everyone else's list, to be true), you need to work on that and reverse the situation. Even if you feel shy, overcome that feeling and reach out to grab your opportunity to shine. Remember that you've got this, so do not let the moment pass you by. Most likely, your date will also feel awkward and uneasy.

Unless she has gone out to a million rendezvous in her life, she will be feeling a little nervous. You should keep that in mind and make sure that she lets go of her shyness gradually, too. But identifying that somebody else is also vulnerable like you can be cathartic. It means that you do not feel isolated and left out. Instead, you address the issue and you realize that you are not the only one experiencing the same thing. Empathy is great, isn't it? I am going to remind you of a classic tip for overcoming anxiety and stress. This is an oldie, but goodie. Whenever you feel overwhelmed by what is going on around you, try to picture all the people without wearing any clothes. In this way, you will have the opportunity to strip them of any superiority they hold over you. If you are thinking of them as more powerful than you, then the game has already been lost. Instead of game over, it is time to swift your mindset and put this strategy to the test.

So next time when you are on a date with a gorgeous girl or right after having approached her to ask for her number, picture her naked. Well, don't get excited, since I am not talking sexually now. Imagine that she does not have any clothes on and therefore she is standing right there, as vulnerable and fragile as you. Consequently, all her secret weapons have gone out of the picture and you can unfold your true intentions, talking to her without sweating from anxiety.

It takes some time to get used to that idea, but it works every single time. You stop thinking of the things that separate you from the person you are talking to and instead you concentrate on the common feeling of vulnerability. Throughout this procedure, you learn how to be stronger and more independent, ultimately relying on yourself. What do you think? Will you keep on shying away from the challenges or will you face them?

Chapter 5:
Acquaintance without Even "Hello"

How many times have you wished that you could communicate with a woman, without even having to say "hello"? Non-verbal communication can be quite intense, since it is straightforward and allows you to fully comprehend what is going on between two people. Is she interested in getting to know you? Is she signaling you to come over and talk to her or is she "speaking out loud" with her body, telling you how amazing she finds you? But getting acquainted seems to follow the same rules every single time, meaning that you ought to build up your confidence and approach her, with the intention to greet her and then see what happens. Or is this not the ONLY way?

Luckily, this is not the only way to meet someone, otherwise it would be so boring and uninspiring. A sequence of events that we would be used to anticipating, without the element of surprise, seems like the wrong way to go! Instead, there are many different options as to how you can start talking to the woman you fancy. In fact, you can make her feel comfortable and intrigue her to come and talk to you. How about that? This would definitely make your day. On top of that, you can talk without even feeling that the conversation has been planned beforehand. Rather than settling for the traditional "hello," you can opt for a variety of situations where you talk to her and she doesn't even question your motive (Whittaker, 2018).

One more thing that you can do to ensure that you get to talk to her, without making the first move verbally, is to make yourself the center of attention. Of course, you need to tread lightly here. You do not want to turn into someone everyone mocks or gossips about. Instead, you should focus on showing her that you are the star within your peer group. You must bring out your alpha male behavior, meaning that you should appear to be powerful and a leader to others. Most women love a leader as their companion, which definitely helps you with your goal. Always check that you come across as gentle and polite, as well. Nobody wants to go out with a savage. Do not get me wrong. I am not claiming here that things can happen like in the movies. I am a grown man and therefore I take pride in avoiding false hopes and high expectations that end up in discomforting situations. But this doesn't mean that you should not give it a go and experiment with your non-verbal skills. In the meantime, you can get her to talk to you without a hitch. How about it?

Getting Her To Take the Lead

How can you attract a woman and make her come and talk to you? As it turns out, your body language will do all the "talking" for you then the rest is up to her. It is true that the way you walk and move around says a lot about who you are and what your intentions are. So if you do not feel comfortable going over there and using a pick-up line that may never work, invite her over with your gestures and attitude. Obviously, you will need to practice this prior to perfecting these skills, but they are so worth it.

First of all, you ought to pay attention to your posture. If your shoulders are in front of your chest and your eyes are constantly looking down, this does not send the right signal as an invitation for a conversation with a beautiful woman. In a similar pattern, if you are always fidgeting and never seem to relax, then this reveals that you are way too nervous to enjoy a laid-back talk with an interesting new acquaintance. And if you avoid eye contact altogether or you keep staring at her, then this can be spooky and off-putting.

You need to appear chilled, casual and confident, friendly and approachable to others - including the woman you want to invite over. Apart from avoiding from bending forward and checking that your shoulders are as wide apart as possible, you should also make sure that you are comfortable. By this, I mean that you ought to get some extra space and show off your coolness, taking up more space than you actually need. Spread your legs so that you look laid back and relaxed. Do the same with your hands and enjoy. This allows you to show your dominance. This is not an excuse for being rude. Therefore, you should not sit down with your feet on a chair or a table. You are trying to impress a woman, not make her dislike you! Start by pushing your shoulders back and keeping your chest clear and wide. This change alone will make a huge difference in the way you look. Not only will it make you appear much fitter and even taller, but it will also allow you to look certain about yourself. Now, in order to keep things light and relaxed, it is essential that you maintain your personal space. In other words, you should not compromise by shrinking into your seat. Instead, set your phone and wallet in front of you, sit back and enjoy your comfort. As far as the eyes are concerned, be strategic. Look her straight into the center of her eyes and when she sees that, do not look away! Smile and then, after a few tiny seconds, look the other way. She will get the signal, trust me. Frankly, body language can go a long way and help you convey messages that you could not send out under other conditions. Still, this is not the only option for you to talk to her without embarrassing yourself or feeling uneasy. In other words, you can find some original ways that make your discussion a necessity, rather than a conscious choice of yours to approach her. I call these methods "lucky encounters", since they appear to rely heavily on the luck factor.

Lucky Encounters

In case you do not want to count on her coming over to talk to you, there are several other tricks up your sleeve. For instance, you can mistake her for the waitress. So rather than hoping that she notices you, it is in your hands to talk to her about your order. "Excuse me, miss, can I order now?" or something like that will surely do the trick. When she tells you that she does not work there, you can both have a laugh and proceed with the rest of the conversation. Another option would be for you to spill some water on her by accident. Yes, this sounds risky and it is, so please do not use anything else but plain water. You do not want her worrying about how to clean that persistent stain off her favorite clothes, right? Of course, this way you could offer to take her clothes to the dry cleaner's, but still with a slight misstep and you can stumble, drenching her with water. "Oh, I am so terribly sorry!" then you watch her reaction. If she is mad, then it is not your day!

Do you find that interesting? A slight variation would be to ask something that makes her feel that her answer matters. For instance, a question that never fails and you do not even have to back up would be "Excuse me, have you seen a tall guy wearing a black hoodie? Has he walked by?" or "Have you noticed any blonde girl in a pink sweater passing by?" Obviously, you need to have some story in the back of your mind to explain who these people are. And please, don't say that you have made that up, as being lied to before the first date is not something any woman would appreciate. Alternatively, you can ask for directions if you are out in the street and you see her from a distance. "Sorry, how can I get to the nearest grocery store?" or whatever, always maintaining the body language signs that have been discussed earlier. If she is sweet and caring, she will most likely try to help you out by giving you directions. Then, the ball is in your court and you had better make great use of that advantage! And of course, you need to work with your surroundings. If you are at a concert, why don't you go and ask her about the latest song that you have just enjoyed? "Are you a fan of this band? Me too!" would also be an acceptable line, lighting the spark for a wonderful conversation.

In general, practice your conversational skills and do not stop until you feel fluent enough to undertake any discussion topic. Clearly, these skills will not only assist you in your struggle to seduce her in time. They will accompany you in your life, making you a more successful professional and facilitating communication with your peers and everyone around you.

Chapter 6:
Be a Nightingale

Everything seems to be heading towards the right direction. You have used my advice and started talking with that lovely woman. Now, after having introduced yourself, greeted her and laid on some compliments, how do you keep that conversation flowing? It seems like a nightmare, not knowing what to say during this silent moment when neither of you talks; it feels like it will last for a lifetime. Will you linger forever in anxiety, doubt and fear? No, I don't think so! It is best that you have planned a whole conversation that enables you to bring up new topics, stimulating a response and prolonging the discussion between you two lovebirds.

Nevertheless, when you talk you are always exposed to reactions to what you are saying. This can backfire and indeed does quite often! As a result, even the most promising conversation is at risk of ending in disappointment. This is why you must know what you are allowed to say, what you must add to your lines and what you should avoid like the plague. One might think that the easiest way to prevent an epic failure would be to talk less and listen more. Well, this is true but on the other hand, how can you promote yourself and reveal your awesomeness if you remain mute? Be a nightingale and keep that conversation flowing effortlessly. Do not be afraid to reveal things about yourself that you know will impress her. If your career has advanced to a point that makes you proud, why shouldn't you say something about it? There is nothing wrong in gloating about your accomplishments, as long as you balance it out and do not come across as a snob. Sure, being the head of a department and supervising a bunch of talented professionals can be challenging and good for you! But seriously, take it down a notch and let her react to what you just said. Prestige is a turn-on to most women, but keep a rather low profile, only scratching the surface of all the amazing things you do daily at work. If she loves it, then you can go on and on with more elaborate details. Until then, hold your horses and wait!

In order to perfect your conversational skills and make the most out of your every word, you should practice. I am sure that you could all use some improvement and it is only fair that you try and try again, before you accomplish perfection. This is why you should take advantage of every single opportunity you get to talk to women of different backgrounds: women of all ages and educational backgrounds, women that you meet on the street or those that you interact with, even briefly. But above anything else, you ought to build up your courage and talk to women that seemingly scare you off. There are intimidating women out there, so you must practice. Start slowly and experiment with different cues. Instead of ordering online, call the store and place that order over the phone, while talking to that helpful employee. Take time to greet the girl that prepares your morning coffee and ask for help at the supermarket. As time passes by and you become more skillful, elevate your game and go for more demanding tasks regarding conversation with women.

Moving forward, you should remember something fundamental. In a discussion with a woman that you like, you should not play it a know-it-all. If you do not know something, do not act like you do simply to impress her. In fact, she will appreciate it a lot more to see that you do not mind admitting that you do not know the answer or that you are clueless about a specific field of interest. Nobody is expected to know EVERYTHING, except Google maybe! So if she talks about a subject that you know absolutely nothing about, let her know. Ask for details. This is a wonderful way to make that conversation flowing naturally.

Things Better Left Unsaid

First off, let's find out what you had better avoid as conversation topics. Some of them are easy to understand why you would dodge them, while others may come as a surprise. Obviously, no woman wants to hear the following line during a pleasant conversation: "Hmm, you are so beautiful. How come you are still single?" This does not serve as a compliment. It is insulting to most women, because they feel like they are being judged for being single. You can compliment her, by all means. Just don't add that last bit. She can be single for a number of reasons, as are you. Judgment and distrust can bring out a truly awkward situation. Besides, there are many people out there still searching for the one or others that do not believe in long-term relationships, marriage and commitment. Asking about previous relationships is a huge no-no, too. Even if she seems cool about it, why scratch an old wound. Why would you ever want to bring it up? This is insane. It is almost as if you were asking her about wanting to have children or if she is close to her parents. These are far too personal questions and they should only be included in a conversation after quite a few dates. More than that, when you ask a woman about her exes, you get to compare with them by default. Why on Earth would you want to do that? It is good that you feel eager to learn more details about her life. However, do not bring up former relationships unless she does.
Remember when I told you not to come across as a snob? Well, this is directly associated with your need to reflect wealth and prestige. There is a thin line that you had better not cross in this case. I am aware that many women find affluence attractive. In fact, some of them spot rich men with their powerful radar and target them. Nonetheless, this does not mean that they are all craving to know more about how wealthy you are. Especially in

the beginning of an acquaintance, insisting on bringing up your financial status might give the wrong impression. You are not trying to bribe her, are you?

Politics must be kept off as a topic, which I know is a no-brainer. Who wants to fight over the best president or prime minister of all time? Healthcare, social insurance and benefits do not sound appealing and are surely not going to advance the conversation in a fruitful manner. There are topics that promote heated conversation, but not in a constructive manner. They are more prone to fueling fights and disputes so you must make sure that you do not mention anything too provocative, at least on your first date.

In general, try to focus on something less controversial that will keep the conversation interesting, without provoking sentiments or raising too many questions. This is exactly why you need to prepare yourself and keep some easy, light and to-the-point topics ready in your arsenal. You never know when they will come in handy!

I know that silence can be awkward for both of you, so there is an urge to cover all these pauses of your conversation with topics. Nevertheless, this is not always true. Sometimes, you really need a minute or two to take in all the things you have been talking about. Do not get uncomfortable every time there is a small pause. Embrace it and appreciate the fact that you both feel confident enough to allow these moments of silence. Otherwise, you would be sweating with anxiety to talk about random stuff, just to fill the void. Up to a point, silence should not be considered a bad thing; instead, it should be regarded as beneficial to the conversation itself.

Don't Be Boring

Let's face it, most people overestimate their conversational skills. They think that they can talk to everybody effortlessly, modifying their methods to match each person's interests. What they do is use some topics that lack originality, simply because they allow them to continue on talking. But this is not the right way to go.

A woman rarely wants to go out with the man that has made her yawn from boredom! So you need to weave some delightful details into your lines, aiming to make you stand out from the crowd. It doesn't take rocket science to understand that asking her to tell you about herself is too generic. Instead, you should get creative and ask something like "I bet your life is exciting. Tell me, what do you do for a living?" or "How do you relax, after an intense day at work?" These questions do not only serve as absolute ice breakers, but they also give her the opportunity to be under the spotlight and lead the conversation precisely where she wants it to go.

After getting to know her, play with the answers that she has already given you. This is a true treasure chest, assuming that you know how to appreciate hidden gems once you find them. If you realize that she is into a sport or hobby, ask more about that but in an eventful way. "I had no idea patchwork could be that fun. What is it about it that excites you?" or "Where would the perfect hike take place?" "Are you a Disney fan?" or "If you were stuck in an elevator, who would you rather be with and why?" are great topics that any woman would love to answer. Her work is another no-brainer. "What is it that you love most about your job?" or "What exactly does a chiropractor do and how come you decided to pursue such a profession?" "What made you apply for this job?" and "Tell me, are you a corner office kind of girl or not?" will most probably help you with advancing the conversation. It goes without even saying that you need to listen to how she replies, so that you know if you are on the right track or your radar has to be readjusted accordingly.

Now take notes and listen to what I am about to tell you.

There is a technique that never fails, when you want to ramp up the conversation with a woman that you want to have sex with. This technique is called active listening and it is very simple to implement. Nonetheless, it makes a huge difference in the way the woman feels towards you. In this scenario, you simply let her do the talking. But be careful not to ignore what she is saying, because this would be a nightmare and you will not be able to bounce back unless you listen attentively. Instead, absorb all the things that she is saying. Even the trivial details matter. Now, next is the most crucial part that makes the technique work. Later on in the conversation, you should ensure that you bring up something that she had talked about. Follow up and ask her about it, comment on that topic or say that her story reminded you of something similar. In this way, she will realize that you have been paying attention. Congratulations, you have just earned yourself some points!

The surroundings play an important role, when it comes to picking the right topic for discussion. If you are hiking, you can talk about nature. On the contrary, when walking by the beach you can bring up water sports that you have always wanted to try and ask her if she feels the same way. Obviously, your personal experiences might also do the trick and allow you to share more intimate insights about each other. Do not be afraid of using self-deprecation. Life is too short to be boring, so laugh out loud and make fun of situations that you know are hilarious. Chances are that she will appreciate a man with a great sense of humor.

I have gathered some extra topics that you can talk about, to avoid long pauses that stress you out while you wonder if she is having a good time or not:

"What are your weekends like?"

"What was the most difficult thing that you have ever done?"

"What is in your bucket list?"

"What's your favorite movie in the entire world?"

"Do you enjoy cooking? If so, do you stick to the recipe or go with your gut?"

"What would be a perfect day for you?"

"Are you a city girl or do you prefer outdoors?"

These are all questions that you can safely keep in your notebook. Whenever you feel like you are stuck and need something to fuel that conversation again, feel free to use them. Once she responds, you can play off her words and keep the focus on her until she turns it back to you. Either way, you will have come one step closer to intimacy with her.

Chapter 7:
Ready or Not

Imagine that everything has gone according to plan and the conversation is flowing smoothly. You both seem to enjoy each other's company, laughing, drinking and having fun. Now, is this enough for you to distinguish if the woman in front of you wants to get intimate? How do you know if she is open to having sex with you or she simply needs more time? Yes, you have guessed it right. Things are hardly ever black and white in these situations and you need to focus on the signals that she is sending you. They will be subtle, yet they will let you know what her intentions are for the night.

Men and women are quite different, when it comes to sex. And even though times have changed, slut shaming is a thing and it prevents women from truly liberating themselves. It is true that even nowadays a woman that chooses to be open and ex-periment sexually is not seen like the perfect fit for certain men. This does not do women any justice, since we are talking about human nature and the desire to experience pleasure. When a man wants to have sex, he is typically open and sincere about it. A woman must hold back a little, avoiding being characterized as "too easy." More than that, women often experience emotions differently to men and this makes them less prone to relax and appreciate the moment, with disregard to what others think. So it is quite clear that women will try to hide what they are feeling as much as they can and as elaborately as they can. They will rarely confront you face to face and tell you that they want to go to bed with you. Nevertheless, even if a woman does not want to let her guard down and reveal what she thinks of you sexually, there are several hints that she is sending out through her body language. When she talks to you, when she listens to your voice, when she leans to come closer and when she flirts distinctly without using any words, things can get intense and clear the way for you to jump right in. To be honest, this is the type of language I love most!

Body Signals Always Tell the Truth

Our body never lies, which is why you ought to concentrate on the signals she is sending you. Decode them and you will see if you are having sex tonight or not. One of the most common things that she can do is touch you, subtly and almost unintentionally. By promoting physical contact, she is clearly sending a message that she is open to more intimacy. In fact, she is trying out your boundaries and checking hers at the same time. Obviously, this touching is not going to start out as much, but it is going to intensify gradually. So if you feel her fingers touching your hand and moving all the way to your arm and shoulders, you know you have an opening.
Similarly, she can lean towards you and reveal her breast line. If you are standing up, maybe she touches you with her breasts for a brief moment, until she leans back for a while. This is all a test for you, so that she can see if you are interested in getting closer. Another thing that a woman does to show her attraction and seek more private moments is to reveal her neck, throw back her hair with a decisive move and spread those pheromones, just as mentioned earlier in the book. Body language is a great way to send out even the most provocative messages without realizing what you have done. Still, you will be out there interpreting those signs as you plan to make your move.

It is needless to state the fact that your advancement should go slow and only if you see that she welcomes your behavior. For instance, you have checked her out as she was gently caressing your arm and touching your neck, below your ears and even your chest. Those are straightforward signs that she is seeking something physical. Now it is your turn. Make your move and see how she reacts. Touch her skin and let your fingers wander, until she appears to hold back. If she doesn't, then you are both ready to take it to the next step. Otherwise, relish those moments of slowly discovering her limits.

Obviously, besides her body language, there are also verbal signs to look out for. She may suggest spending time at her place. This is one of the most direct messages to send out, inviting you to take the lead and move forward with a more intimate encounter. Furthermore, the way she talks reveals a lot as to whether or not she is ready to go to bed with you. She will be talking more softly and deeply. Perhaps she sighs every now and then. But the most frequently used weapon a woman engages in is her choice of words while flirting. If she wants you sexually, she will select the proper words to let you know. This will be in the form of innuendos and direct hints, until she eventually expresses her consent and gives you the green light to dive right in (Van Edwards, 2013).

What If She Needs More Time?

Not all women are ready to have sex on the first date. I know, it's a bummer. This is absolutely normal and it does not mean that she doesn't want you sexually. Interpret the signs when you see her holding back, even though she clearly wants you, be the bigger man and give her some space. As a result, she will end up craving your touch even more than before. It is a great thing to show respect to her needs, understanding her insecurities and going above and beyond towards making her feel comfortable. Remember, this is a marathon race and you have not made it to the finish line yet. She may be asking for more time because she wants to test you.

Seduction club

Perhaps she wants to see if you can step up to the plate and take action. It is good to keep that under advisement and avoid any misunderstanding. You need to be quite clear about your intentions. Without putting any pressure on her, go ahead and show her that you are open to more intimacy. Being bold and open while allowing her to breathe and take in what is happening seems like the perfect balance. Try to achieve that and watch the magic as it unfolds before your eyes. She will understand that you respect her needs and at the same time you are brave enough to show her what you need. This will make her feel more comfortable and closer to you, increasing the possibility of her trusting you. Apart from everything that has been discussed so far, it is useful to become conscious of a woman's timeframe. Based on what she believes, her sex tolerance will vary a great deal. There are women out there that do not mind having sex with a man, without even the slightest emotional investment. As a consequence, when you meet such a woman you will find her exceptionally open to having sex with you. Yet, these women will most probably be emotionally unavailable and this is a risk that you have to take. When a woman follows her primal urges and does not take other details into consideration, it makes sense that she is not looking for anything other than sexual pleasure. This is great, if this is solely what you are after. When asking for more time, though, she wants to weigh the pros and cons, showing that at least she cares. You may end up making out, which can be equally satisfying. At least, you will realize that her sexual interest is real, making things promising for the next date. Your task is to help her overcome her fears and see that you are for real. It is in your hands to allow her to let go of her hesitation and indulge in absolute pleasure. You have all the time in the world to show her that sex will only elevate your relationship and offer you both what you are entitled to. Do not forget that many women have been raised under the impression that you should NOT have sex before the third date. Until then, be sure to show her that sex is not the only reason you are talking to her, spending time with her and making plans for a date. And frankly, it shouldn't be.

Chapter 8:
Best Places to Meet

Congratulations! You have made it halfway through the book. I am sure that you have already acquired precious knowledge that allows you to reach your goal to seduce a woman in seven hours tops. In order to perfect your skills, though, and become a seductive sex machine, keep reading. I will let you know exactly how to use all this information to your advantage, luring women into your irresistible weave and making them crave your love. Wouldn't that be something?

We have already discussed the best places to go on a date, as well as some places that you should avoid. But now it is time to think about a different aspect. What happens when you meet a woman that you like and want to take her on a date. Now, time is ticking and you should prepare for your next move. But what will it be? Should you suggest going on a date at the same time, on the spot? Or maybe it would be best to schedule your date for the next day or the weekend ahead?

I am pretty sure that your impulse would be to go ahead and spend time with her right then and there. And this is a wonderful feeling, to begin with. However, this is not always the best piece of advice. There are many factors that determine whether or not you should wait. These important variables will help you understand if you should suggest continuing on with your date right away or call it a day and schedule something else soon. For example, where have you met her? What time of day is it? Where are you heading? What is the weather like? All these questions will probably enlighten you as to what to do.

Remember that you should not let emotions or impulses get the best of you. For instance, you might run into her on your way to the dentist's. It makes absolutely no sense to invite her over, as you open your mouth widely to have your wisdom tooth pulled out. Nor should you schedule a date in the same evening, with the anesthesia still kicking in and preventing you from pronouncing words properly. You might think that I am exaggerating and you are probably right. Yet, you should take this advice and use it as a guideline for your upcoming experiences. Even if you meet her at the supermarket, do you think that she will be over the moon if you suggest ditching groceries to grab a cup of coffee?

How to Play It Out

In this section, I am going to show you some meeting options and how you should adapt, depending on where and when you meet. Firstly, what if you just met in the street? It is morning, you have just grabbed your morning fix (a freshly brewed coffee) and you are on your way to work, when you see a gorgeous creature. You manage to talk to her and she is clearly giving you a positive vibe. Well, even though you would really love to proceed with a date strolling around the city and talking about anything, just to listen to her voice, compose yourself. All these things you both have to do will hold you back from enjoying your time together, since in the back of your mind you will know that you have tons of obligations just waiting for you. So do yourself a favor and schedule a date with her another time.

When you meet at a bar, things are much simpler. You can have drinks there and see where things are going. A bar has everything it takes, including lounge music, alcohol and a laid-back atmosphere that makes everything more relaxing and cooler. Besides, you might know the barista or the owner there or maybe you have a couple of cool stories to tell her about this place. But if you have already had too much to drink, then you should avoid embarrassing yourself. It is great that you have managed to talk to that beautiful lady, but do not push your luck. Reschedule and be sure to avoid overdrinking, if you really want to enjoy your date. Nobody appreciates drunk people, unless they are members of a fraternity in college.

Time is of the essence, so be careful when you arrange where and when to go out on your date. If you meet early in the afternoon, maybe you can plan your date for later on the same day. You will have enough time to prepare, but also not have to wait too long. Listen to her and work around her schedule, so that she knows that you want to please her. But it is best that you suggest where to meet, in order to reveal your dominant side. In a nutshell, things are quite flexible when it comes to meeting. The most important aspect is to find the specific timing that is convenient for both sides. Given that, you may have to wait a little until you do find something that ticks all the boxes. No worries, this can add to the suspense and allow your desire to grow.

Too Soon or Too Late?

When is the right time to schedule a date? Honestly, I cannot answer that for sure. As mentioned above, there are so many little things that define the best time. But due to this significant flexibility, you may have concerns as to whether or not you will be able to identify the right moment. You would hate to lose the momentum you have built. If you wait too long, you are risking to let that acquaintance slip away. Unless you have made such a great first impression, you cannot expect her to wait patiently until you decide to give her a call. She will most likely focus on someone else, if she hasn't already.

On the other hand, trying to avoid just that can make you end up coming across as needy and insecure. You just met her two hours ago, so how can you not hold it together until tomorrow?

Seduction club

If you cannot discipline yourself, find adequate distractions that keep your mind busy and your fingers away from the phone. Even though I still believe that timing can vary greatly, this does not mean that there is not a minimum timeframe for you to follow. In this case, you must wait at least half a day (so 12 hours) in total until you make your move. Of course, she can always surprise you and take matters into her own hands, supposing she can't wait to see you.

I am sure that you have heard of rules that tell you to avoid calling until at least three days have passed after your first encounter. Some people will claim that you should count backwards from 100, each time you get the urge to send her a text message or give her a call. Others will insist that you have done enough and that it is her turn to show you if she is interested or not. But take it from my personal experience, every acquaintance is entirely different. And this is the beauty of it all! Obviously, there are some steps that facilitate the process of hooking up with the woman that you want.

The bottom line is that you should not worry so much about the timing, as each case is quite unique. If you meet the woman of your dreams and she shares your enthusiasm. Why wait? There is absolutely no rule of thumb here, as long as you both agree on the time and place. Be open and flexible, so that you can work around her schedule and organize a date that is convenient for both of you. Rather than dealing with trivial stuff, such as how long you should wait until you ask her out or until you follow up with a second date, appreciate each moment and make the most out of your experience.

Chapter 9
Give a Call

So you have not gone out on a date yet. However, it is good that you have her number. Normally, you would have called her the minute you lost sight of her. But come on, why do that and ruin all the hard work you have put into this endeavor? Now you need to decide when is the best time to call her, after your initial encounter. On the one hand, you do not want to scare her off. Still, on the other hand you must make sure that she understands that you are indeed interested in her. She is not just a random acquaintance, rather than a woman who has made quite an impression on you.

It has been known forever that the ideal time between getting her number and actually using it should range from two to five days. Nonetheless, you do not have to stick to that rule. The only thing that you need to make sure is that at least 24 hours have passed, since you obtained her phone number. Otherwise, you are giving her the wrong idea. If you get the phone number and call in 15 minutes, then you are sending out the message that you have fallen hopelessly for her or that you are so creepy and cannot discipline yourself. Neither of those options is great. You are not in a hurry.

If you cannot wait for the 24-hour time period, I suggest that you do whatever it takes to make time fly. And at least wait until the next day to call. For instance, if you got her number at the bar last night, then just wait until after midday then make a call. Obviously, there is a chance she misses your call due to being busy or not recognizing the number you are calling from. In that case, this is a different challenge for you. Do not repeat the phone call. Even if she doesn't return your call, do not fall for that trap. Be strict about it, otherwise you can appear too needy. Just wait and she will call you or wait until the next day to try again.

If you appear to be too clingy, by rushing into contacting her right after your first date, this can backfire. You do not want that. Obviously, there are men who overanalyze things and are emotionally prone to lean on a woman from the very beginning. No matter what you may think, most women do not value such behavior. On the contrary, they see it as proof that you are overly needy and this does not leave room for the image of a powerful man with strong will and the desire to dominate. Think about it and change your mindset accordingly, the sooner the better.

What to Say

You have her number, you call her and she picks up! What do you say? Do not overthink this, but be prepared for what you are about to tell her. Have something planned, including how to ask her out and where to take her on your first date. But first, it is crucial that you come across as calm and confident. Talk in a soothing voice, be friendly and pleasant towards her. Of course, you will need to greet her before anything else. A simple "hello" can do the trick. Then, remind her briefly who you are and see how she reacts. If she does not recall your acquaintance, then you had better target a different woman. But by giving you her number, she has probably been expecting that call all day.

Ask her about her day, because otherwise you may sound rude. It is the polite thing to say, after all. Listen to her talk and interpret her words. She is most likely testing you, too. Then, go ahead with suggesting going on a date. Be firm and always keep that friendly tone. "I would love to take you out tonight, what do you say?"

is a great line. It is casual enough and does not put too much pressure on that special lady of yours. Even if she can't, wait for her counter-proposal.

Always keep a backup plan that you can turn to. Maybe she does not like the place you have recommended or she might be too busy to go out with you. This does not mean that she is not interested, that's life! So be sure to offer alternatives. Remember that the clock is ticking, but this only applies to the real interaction time you spend with her. If this week is no good for her and she suggests going out next week, do her a favor! Obviously, if she keeps giving negative responses, then this is an indication that you had better give her some space and let her decide if she wants to go out with you. But under no circumstances should you insist.

A great piece of advice that you should implement not only when meeting a beautiful lady, but also in any other interaction you have with people, is to rationalize. In other words, be realistic as to the gravity of the situation. You are about to talk to a woman, end of story. Your life does not depend on it and you have done it thousands of times before. You do talk to the cashier at the supermarket, the woman that comes over your store to order stuff, as well as many other people every single day. This means that you are an expert as to how to talk to women! Use this expertise to get over any anxiety you may have.

What About Texting Her?

There are many misconceptions about texting a woman after getting her number. Again, there is no one-size-fits-all option. Both choices, calling and texting, come with their pros and cons. Texting is a safer way to contact a woman, especially if you are under 30. Most communication starts out like that and it would be awkward to call her, in that case. But on the other hand, calling lets her know that you are bold and do not shy away from a challenge. It is far more personal and most women get more flattered when they receive a phone call, compared to a text. Throughout a phone call, you can sense if she is happy to listen to you. The tone of her voice, the comments and reactions to everything you say offer invaluable feedback for you as to whether or not you are standing a chance with her.

Texts are great when you have not perfected your talking skills and you still want to impress her. If that happens, you should think of something to write that will make her smile. Maybe a subtle joke or a follow-up on something you have said the night before will definitely let her know that you have been thinking of her. Do not be too lengthy. You are not taking an exam! Still, always pay attention to typos and proper sentence structure. Do not be inelegant, either. "I hope you had a good night's sleep after those appletinis." or "Is that song still on your mind, after last night at the bar?" can be good introductory lines for you to use. But in case you decide to contact her via social media, do not get carried away and check when the message gets delivered and read. If you do, this will only add to your anxiety and fill you with doubts that you certainly do not need right now.

One thing that you need to pay attention to, though, when it comes to texting, is the length. By that, I mean that you should not engage in never-ending conversations with her. If you both enjoy talking to each other, then why not do that face to face? A text is great as an introduction, a prelude to the main course. But it should never replace the main course, because this would set you astray from your end goal. So right after you text her and let her know your number and contact information, be sure to proceed to the next level. Tell her that you would love to meet and hang out together some time. See if she just wants to spend some time texting back and forth or if she is interested in a more private conversation over drinks. Texting is good, but only in terms of fixing a date in person. And as far as size is concerned, the smaller the better. I know it is counter-intuitive, but keep the text simple and easy to comprehend. Don't send anything fancy or overly complicated.

Are you torn between these two choices and you cannot decide? I have the ideal option that will bring out the best of both worlds. You can send her a text, acting as an introduction to a phone call. "Hi there, it's me John from last night. I am sending you this message so that you have my number, too. What time would it be convenient for me to call you?"

This serves as a text, but simultaneously allows you to throw the idea of calling on the table. Now you are expecting her answer, be it in written form or in the form of a phone call. No matter what you do, please do not ask her if she remembers you. This only makes her feel that you do not value yourself enough. Aren't you worthy of being remembered one day after you met? Sure you are, so do not even imply otherwise. Women notice those things and they do not make you look so good.

Chapter 10
Candy-Flower Period

I bet you are a truly giving person, who enjoys watching joy spark in other people's eyes or seeing the way their face lights up. Of course, you are used to offering gifts to those who matter to you. Presents are exciting on so many different levels. But when you have just met a woman that you fancy and want to have sex with, you need to be very careful. First of all, you do not want to seem like you are trying to bribe her. This is not your goal. A present may come across as too forward or even too much. Besides, you do not know her that well so as to know what she enjoys and what she hates. So, what should you do? Avoid gifts altogether or risk getting something that does not hit the spot?

When you make a new romantic acquaintance, you dive into mysterious dark waters where you are expected to show off your swimming skills. Choosing to rise to the challenge of finding the most suitable present will earn you points in her system and this is what you are after. Without engaging in extravagant expenses and gifts that give out the wrong idea about you, you can buy something that she loves and accomplish your goal of impressing her even more.

This is not necessary; so if you are not that kind of guy that offers flowers or thinks of original gifts for his loved ones, then don't worry about it. However, when you give someone a present, you instantly make them smile and believe (even subconsciously) that you have taken the time to think about them. Making her realize that you have been thinking of her will not hurt a bit!

Even if you have spoken for a few minutes, you must have gathered some useful information about her. Try to recall her looks, the way she was dressed, her accessories and so on. All these elements can help you understand what the perfect present would be for her. It should be something that sparks a conversation and makes an impression on her. Even a small accessory for her hair, bath salts or a small organizer might help you get a little closer to her heart. It shows you have put some thought into it and managed to find a correlation as to why you have chosen that present over anything else. And by all means, less is more on this special occasion and therefore you should not go overboard and spend a whole fortune on a present. This is not the right time.

When Is The Right Time?

Should you give her the present yourself on your first date or send it over before you meet? Or maybe wait until the first date is over then send over something, to tell her how lovely the evening was. These are all great options, although you must be careful not to overreact. If you choose to send a present over to her before the date, this should be discreet and cute. After a first date, you can show more passion and reveal your romantic nature. Finally, if you opt for giving the present to that wonderful woman during your date, then you need to be creative. Go for something that you have talked about or buy a present that is funny, sweet, practical and a little "out of the box."

For the ultimate romantic gesture, a bouquet of flowers is always a wonderful gift. In fact, even a single rose can work wonders. Another great option is candy, meaning chocolate! Heart-shaped chocolate candy will send her the message that she is sweet and that she has set out on a journey to your heart, which can be enticing for her! Teddy bears and other cute stuff for her bedroom can also make a good impression, but it depends on her age group and her character.

When it comes to frequency, things are quite strict. You only do that once then you see how it plays out. Thanks to your present, you are direct and you claim her attention. You have made your move and it is time for her to react accordingly. If she likes the gesture, she will make her own move and that will definitely bring her closer to your bed. Otherwise, there is no point in sending her another present.

What about the Color?

Have you ever thought of how the color of your present speaks louder than a thousand words? It makes sense. Why should you focus on what you buy her, not only regarding its material and purpose? You need to pay attention to the color of your gift, since this reveals a lot about your intentions and the feelings that you want to awaken. So even if you have had an epiphany and want to give her flowers, be sure to check below to find out the meaning of each color.

Everybody knows that red is the color of passion and love, energy and desire. It is also the color that represents primal urges. On Valentine's Day, stores decorate their displays with scarlet red hearts and gifts. Red lipstick is the ultimate turn-on for most men and red underwear will turn any woman into a sex machine. Isn't that enough to conclude that you should select red color, if you are after a relationship of passion and intense emotions? You can never go wrong with the classics and red is definitely an all-time classic color for couple gifts.

Blue on the other side is the color of tranquility, healing and inner peace. Its soothing qualities make it an excellent choice, when you want to put someone at ease. Blue tones also reflect the truth and reveal intelligence. This is not a bad option for a gift, but I am not sure that this is the best you can do on a first date. A much better solution would be to opt for green. This is also a healing color, but at the same time comes across as something fresh and in line with nature. The darker the green, the more it correlates with the presence of money and hence you should think twice before selecting such a gift.

Yellow is a cheerful color and promotes happiness, optimism and warmth in emotions. It is a great way to show somebody that you care, without making it too obvious or highlighting your romantic side. Gold is a much more sophisticated option, since it is directly associated with riches and abundance. Therefore, it is ideal for those looking to focus on their prestige. And finally, orange combines the features of red and yellow and is the perfect present to demonstrate enthusiasm and a positive vibe (CK, 2015).

Chapter 11
Come to Me

Your date is working out great so far. You are both in a good mood, you communicate well and it seems like you have hit it off perfectly. Now what? How do you bring up sex? It is true that you are on a tight schedule, considering that you should seduce her in seven hours or less. After all this time of meeting and talking and planning the date, what's next? Should you mention it right away or wait to see what she does instead? And if things are looking so promising right now, why not take a risk and see how it plays out? It is true that men can put women under pressure when it comes to sex. This happens because they are driven directly by their urges and they want to satisfy their needs. There is nothing wrong with that, by the way. However, in order to achieve your goals and have sex on the first date, you need to be smart and plan ahead. As always, there is no guarantee that she will agree to proceed with intercourse. But through these carefully planned moves, you increase your chances and come closer to her, one way or another. Beware not to force things, because nothing good has ever come out of such behavioral patterns. Instead, there is always the risk of scaring her off and making her feel uncomfortable. So it is essential that you avoid such behavior that puts her on edge. Think of it like a game of chess. Do not waste your moves, always interpreting the re-actions of your opponent and trying to be one step ahead. Of course, your date should not be considered an enemy but you get the gist!

If she feels nervous about the possibility of having sex, then you don't stand a chance. She will bail on you sooner or later. Or else, she will try to overcome her fears and this frequently ends up in drinking too much to build up the courage she needs to get on with this. Even if she doesn't drink, she will rush into sex then she may feel guilty, spoiling all the fun. It is human nature and, to be more accurate, female nature to do that. So make sure that her consent is real and indisputable, unless you are up for that roller-coaster of emotions.

Now, let's get back to business. You have weighed the pros and cons and you are ready to ask her to continue your date back home. From the signals you have caught onto, she is clearly feeling it too and you will have a blast in bed. In theory, you have worked things out perfectly. Practice, however, seems to be a little trickier than what you would have hoped. So how do you ask her to come over? Do you let her make the first move or do you jump right in?

Asking Her to Come Over: When and How

It is important to evaluate the situation, before asking her to come over to your place for some "alone time". Throughout your date, you should have started assessing where you are at. For example, even upon meeting you ought to establish some sort of physi-cal contact. I am not talking about anything inappropriate, just basic stuff that will help you break the ice and come closer. Hug her and give her a swift kiss on the cheeks, checking out how she responds to this level of intimacy. When you talk, touch her occasionally to gauge if she is feeling nervous or comfortable. And as I have mentioned earlier, read between the lines to com-prehend what her body language is telling you. When you feel confident enough, proceed with caution and notice her reactions. The best way to do that is by suggesting to go over to your place for a while, leaving her the option to leave as soon as she gets agitated or feels that it is not fun for her any more. As a result, the woman will know that she has the upper hand and it is her choice to stay or leave. This way, she will feel more comfortable and she will have the opportunity to relax and enjoy the moment. "Shall we go to my place for a while? You can leave when you want to, so what do you think?" is a great way to introduce the option of sex to her, letting her decide. "I guess we could continue our conversation at my place, maybe get a drink or two. Are you up for this?" is also good. Do not be abrupt and please take "no" for an answer if that is what she says.

According to her response, you can tell if you are having sex or not. When a woman follows you home after a date, it means that she wants to go the extra mile. But even then, it is a matter of balancing her doubts and fears with her desire to have sex. Be gentle and polite at all times, leaving her some breathing room and offering her the freedom to choose what she does next. It is amazing to show off your dominant side, maintaining at the same time your polite nature and your flexibility as per her own desires and preferences.

It goes without even saying that your place needs to be clean and tidy before bringing your date there. Otherwise, your chances of getting laid will drop significantly. A huge mess is one of the major turn-offs for women, so be careful and do not fall for that. Dedicate some time to fold your clothes and tuck them away, clean up the toilet and wash the dishes. Do not go overboard, but make sure that she knows you are clean, responsible and pro-hygiene. Another thing to keep in mind is that you must never, under any circumstances, be direct about sex verbally. "Shall we fuck?" is a disaster and no woman appreciates such abrupt suggestions, even if she indeed wants to get some. So restrain your urges for total sincerity and go slow. Use your body language and pay her compliments, making her feel wanted. Since she is at your place after a date, she clearly wants you. Build on your moves gradually, touching her while you are making out and eventually trying to unbutton her shirt or something. Then, always see how she reacts. If she is feeling good, go on and enjoy!

In this way, if you learn how to pace yourself and wait a little until you get to the bottom step and ask her to come in, you increase your chances of succeeding. As a result, you slowly build sexual tension and you let her come to the point where she cannot say "no." Flirting with her but still allowing her to give permission take that next step will lead to an explosion of lust. You say something sexy and then follow up with a comment about something entirely different; go on like this and you will see her transform into a sex goddess calling out your name!

What If She Says No

It is not the end of the world, man. OK, it is a bummer to suggest going over at your place for sex and having her turn you down. But this does not mean that you are going to stop trying. In fact, this can be a great challenge and hence you should appreciate the fact that she is making you work for it. After rejecting you, she will most likely want to see how you react. Do not appear to be bitter or angry about what just happened. On the other hand, you should not give up. Your best bet is to persist in building the perfect sexy ambiance and making her want you so much that she cannot resist any longer next time you get together.

When a woman does not come by your house after a date, maybe she needs more time or she is intimidated by you. Or she might think it is too soon for you to spend time alone, without first having learned a few more things about each other. Follow her lead and show that you are there for her, listening to what she wants and needs. However, respect her decision to say "no" and do not hold her accountable for that. It is not necessary for the first date to end in sex. What is important is that you build the foundations for sex, even if it means to wait for a little bit until you follow up.

Again, the situation here can be very fluid. If she looks offended when she refuses going back to your place, obviously this is a clear sign that she is not into you.

Chapter 12
She Said "Yes"

That escalated fast, right? You are out on a date, enjoying your time together and feeling sexual tension. It is perfectly clear that you are both ready to take things to the next level. But there is always the fear of rejection. So you wait and wait and then, finally, you get that precious confidence boost that allows you to spell it out for her. "Do you want to come over to my place for more privacy?" then she says "Yes." It seems that your luck has changed! Although this has nothing to do with luck, to be honest. You have been preparing yourself all this time, so that you know how to behave and follow what steps will drive you to this end result. Nonetheless, you are not off the hook just yet.

Upon hearing the magic words from her luscious mouth that you want to kiss and lick and bite so much, what do you do next? If you are out in a bar, do you ask for the bill before she even gets the chance to finish her drink or do you wait? Obviously, you do not want to let the moment fade away and miss your chance. Even though the woman has agreed to go home with you, it does not mean that she will be thinking the same thing after an hour or so. Women tend to overthink things, so this means that she will be spending the next hour trying to consider all the negative consequences of her agreement to follow you home. All that second guessing does not help you reach your goal and you know that. However, it is crucial that you do not come across as overly enthusiastic about her decision. Consequently, you need to wait a little until you confirm going back home with her and continuing on with your game of seduction. Finish your drinks or, if your glasses are empty, order another cocktail or a couple of shots. Talk for a while, even for a few minutes, then ask the waiter for the bill. In this way, you show her that you've got this. You have everything under control. Evidently, you do not need to mask your content for her assent to visit your home. Otherwise, you would be competing for the Oscars!

My Place or Yours?

This is another important element that should be discussed. Should you invite her over to your place and insist on going there? Or should you be open to her counter-suggestion to visit her home instead? Well, there are advantages and disadvantages in either of these options. Your place is your kingdom and you will be feeling 100 percent in control of your surroundings. It is your shelter, so your prey ought to follow you there. Plus, you have been cleaning all day making sure that everything is great, so why not get credit for that? Maybe you have bought a champagne for the occasion, along with some scented candles and a few chocolate treats. You must be rewarded for your preparedness, right?
On the other hand, when you go by her place, she will immediately feel more comfortable. As a result, she will have fewer doubts about having sex with you. Her bedroom is safe in her eyes and she will most probably drop her inhibitions. More than that, when you go by her house you can learn a lot about her and of course you will not be judged as to the state of your own home. She will not spend time observing your furniture and the way you stack your clothes, nor will she second guess if you have cleaned the bathroom or changed the bed sheets.
Her home is the last frontier that you will need to conquer.
So if she insists that you go there rather than your place, think of yourself as a warrior in battle. You can take up this challenge too. Do anything to make her feel at ease and take those worries off

her mind. After all, you both have a lot on your plate and you had better concentrate on more pleasurable things.

Of course, desperate times call for desperate measures. I am only joking, but there is something that you may have not considered enough yet. She might not have availability to take you back to her place and yours might not be ideal. There are millions of reasons why, including a nosy roommate or lack of time to clean up, or the presence of skeletons in the closet and so on. For all these reasons, you must have a backup plan as to where to get intimate. In most cases, a hotel offers great accommodation for shorter or longer time periods.

I know, a hotel is hardly a place that you would call romantic or fitting for your first time sex. But when there is no other alternative that works for both of you, should you let the opportunity pass you by? No way. In fact, a hotel may be proven the perfect place for hot and steamy sex. It is clean and goal-oriented, meaning that the bed is indeed the centerpiece of the room and there is a fully functional bathroom right there. Clean sheets, comfy pillows, air conditioning and extra amenities that you can both use elevate the experience. Just be sure you know you are heading to a quality establishment, in avoidance of disastrous situations. You don't want a mattress infested with bed bugs ruining the moment, do you?

A hotel can be great for another reason, too. It is a neutral ground, so nobody feels left out or uneasy. So this means that you can both relax and enjoy intimate moments of pleasure, without worrying about practical stuff like if she is going to notice the pile of dirty dishes in the kitchen. And she is not going to have concerns like whether or not the neighbors saw you two getting in the house. Plus, hotels are the absolute epitome of sexual fantasies.

The Perfect Time Is Now

Some people get carried away by their desire to control all things during a crucial moment like this one. Although it is good to be prepared and improve your odds of success, you need to take it easy and not beat yourself up if things do not go as planned. She has said "yes" and this is a solid reason to celebrate. Now, the conditions play an important role, but they are not vital as to the outcome of your date. Instead of focusing on what has not gone according to your initial plan, why don't you try to appreciate how far you have become? This is going to be your night, filled with passion and pleasure. So don't even think about regrets.

When you fantasize about something, you structure even the slightest detail and expect things to go a certain way. But then reality kicks in and you see that things never go exactly as planned. Maybe a line you wanted to use never came up, since you have been busy talking about other topics. Or perhaps you have been anticipating coming back to your home later and she kept saying that she preferred her place. The list goes on and on. Still, there is no room for disappointment. Things have played out great so far and now you are on your way to her bed sheets, which will probably smell and feel much better than yours!

The perfect time is now. The perfect place is where you are with her and this is what you should concentrate on. Enjoy the moments you spend together, treasure them and do your best to make this night memorable. Even though there will always be trivial changes to the plan that you have thought over again and again, the truth is that the plan has taken you all the way to here. So cherish the plan and do not just think that it has not served its purpose to the fullest. Because it has.

Chapter 13
Do Not Screw Up

Things are getting serious. You are alone with the woman that has been haunting your dreams and fantasies. This is the moment you have been hoping for and you need to live up to her expectations. If you fail, then neither of you will want to remember anything about this night. But if you succeed, then this can be a remarkable experience for both of you. And who knows? Maybe seducing her in less than seven hours does not end with plain sex. At least, it might be the beginning of more and more sex along the way. So it is essential that you do not screw up at this stage. An opportunity like this should not be underestimated. Again, I urge you to consider all the details beforehand. If you are inviting a woman over to your home, you must have first analyzed all the options and have everything taken care of to the slightest little detail. Your home ought to be a reflection of yourself, so you should take the time to make it spotlessly clean and add some personal touches of awesomeness to its style. Then, you must buy all the supplies that may come in handy during your stay with her. A bottle of wine, chilling in the fridge, along with some simple yet delicious treats, will do the trick. Cute glasses, comfy pillows and clean sheets, a shiny bathroom with fresh towels, all these elements will add to her feeling at ease. And this is what you should be looking forward to.

I might sound abrupt, but trust me on this. You should not leave any room for failure. Even though it might seem that you are going to score 100 percent, this is far from the truth. Within just a fragment of a second, all your hard work may go to waste due to some unimportant minor detail. So double your vigilance and remain calm, bold and daring to ensure her indisputable seduction. It all starts with her feeling comfortable, cozy and safe.

Making Her Feel at Ease

So you just entered the apartment, you invited her in and turned on the lights. She starts wandering around with her eyes and your main goal is to make her feel comfortable. So what do you do? First of all, you tell her to sit down wherever she wants. In this way, you give her the freedom to choose where she feels less threatened. It makes sense, when somebody is not familiar with a specific place, to take some time before they feel welcome and relaxed. By selecting where she sits, she gains some sort of control over the room and this is soothing for her.

Of course, you can also give her the tour to your home. This is another thing that is going to calm her down. As a result, she will know what to expect when you move on to the bedroom from the living room and she will be more comfortable to find and use the bathroom. These are small details that a man hardly ever pays attention to. Women are quite different, though. So allow her to get acquainted with the place until she lets her guard down.

Soft, lounge music is great to feel romantic and get in the mood for some sweet loving. Even before leaving home for your date, you should prepare a playlist with several songs that will make both of you more prone to romance. Obviously, this is not the time for death metal or folk songs. Be realistic and think of the songs you love listening to, when you get intimate. Aim for music that awakens the senses and gives you goosebumps. Light some scented candles, as the aroma will be intoxicating and can help you both relax.

Get that wine or champagne out of the fridge, serve it chilled in clean glasses and sit by her side. Make a toast (nothing fancy or time-consuming, a simple "To us" would suffice) and take the first sip, before kissing her on the lips. But since you are in your personal territory, give her some time to follow your lead and do not claim her space. She always needs to feel comfortable and calm.

As for small talk, it doesn't really matter what you say, as long as you say something. The tone of your voice should remain soothing and bold at the same time. You are daring and focused, which is exactly how you want her to see you, rather than insecure or doubtful. Pay her a compliment or two, whisper sweet words in her ear and breathe slowly, as you are getting closer and closer to her. Take your time, go really slowly and dance to her rhythm.

Out of Your Comfort Zone

Alternatively, you will go back to her place. So any effort you have made as to how to control your surroundings has now gone to waste. But this should not add any frustration or anxiety to your evening. Besides, she invited you over and this means that she wants to get more intimate. Just make sure that you familiarize yourself with her place from the moment you set your foot in. Check out where everything is placed, spot the bathroom and the bedroom and show respect. This means that you should not throw yourself on the sofa and lay back with your feet on the coffee table. Compliment her on her choice of artwork or color scheme. Be sure to ask for permission to use the bathroom. Of course she will say yes, but it is common courtesy and you must play along.

Being at her place definitely means that you are somewhat out of your comfort zone. You cannot light the candles, bring the wine out for a romantic toast or get some lounge music playing in the background. However, think of it the other way around.

You just sit there and wait to be pampered. She needs to get you feel comfy and at ease, isn't this great? Enjoy her care and hospitality, while maintaining your politeness and you are on the right track. Obviously, you may need to comply with some special requirements of hers, such as taking your shoes off before entering the apartment or using a certain bathroom. There is nothing wrong with that, so deal with it. And if you are a smoker, think twice before lighting that cigarette or vaping. Assuming that it is impossible to resist, always ask for permission and ensure that you are as discreet as you can be.

The whole point is that you must think outside the box and increase your flexibility as to where you are feeling comfortable. Things hardly ever go exactly as planned, which is what you need to accept, before moving forward. This book will hopefully help you with several different aspects of female seduction. From now on, you know how to deal with various situations and make the most out of your potential. Yet, life is unpredictable and you should be well aware of that. Therefore, do not stick rigidly to the rules, instead be ready to bend them accordingly. Under no circumstances should you fear getting out of your comfort zone. Rather, revel in expanding your comfort zone!

Chapter 14

What about the Socks?

Are ready to have sex? You are feeling very confident by now. So after having followed my advice as to how to approach a woman, make an interesting acquaintance and getting her number, scheduling to go out on a first date and then going back either at your place or hers, it is safe to say that you are on your way to having sex. I am guessing it took you about seven hours to achieve those goals. Now, it is time to enjoy the main course of your hard training and you should be prepared for what is about to happen. To make a great impression (since first impressions matter), you need to be goal-oriented and make sure that you have got everything covered.

Before meeting her, you should buy proper protection. There is no room for negligence in this aspect. It is a huge turn off for a woman to realize that the man she is making out with has not acted prudently enough to buy condoms. Other than that, you need to pay attention to your outfit. This means that you ought to double check your underwear and socks, which can either make or break the entire experience. And of course, it is needless to say that all apparel must be perfectly clean and in good condition. No stretched boxers or socks with holes on them will do. And for the love of God, check your shoes - if they give out any funny smell, choose a different pair!

Impeccable personal hygiene is a given. There should be no objection about that. Take time for a leisurely shower that allows you not only to relax, but also to look spotlessly clean and sharp. Choose your favorite clothes, the ones that make you feel hot. This is what you are after, isn't it? A shirt ironed to perfection and giving away the shape of your abs is great. However, you can wear anything you like, as long as you feel good the way you are dressed. After all, you must ooze with confidence and the proper outfit will assist you in that. Moreover, you can use that wonderful cologne that your mum bought you for your birthday or at least use aftershave. Now is the time to do it!

Moving on to the fun part, sex typically means that you both take your clothes off. But what do you do? Do you wait for her to get undressed and undress you too or do you take charge? It would be good to try first to unzip her pants or unbutton her shirt to see how she reacts. Maybe she likes that kind of initiative or she would rather do it herself. Go with whatever pleases her. Similarly, give her some time to see if she reaches for your pants and, if not, then get naked on your own. Remember that anticipation enhances desire and hence you should take it slow, not rushing into things and definitely giving yourself some time before getting fully naked.

Yes, fully naked means that you will need to take your socks off, too. Unless it is freezing cold, there is no other excuse why you should leave them on. Or if you choose to indulge in some steamy, intense sex making while standing up and removing only what is absolutely necessary. In that case, you can get away with that. But wait a minute. Is standing up the perfect position for first time sex?

Best Place for First Time Sex

When you think of having sex, the first thing that comes to mind is definitely the bedroom. Lying on the mattress, cuddling with your partner under the bed sheets and with the comfy pillows.

Seduction club

This is a wonderful option for enjoying sex with your new partner. You will both feel comfortable, since this is the traditional place where sex magic happens. And it will allow you to experiment with different sex positions, as the bed is typically spacious enough for you to twist and turn. In this case, you can start with the missionary position and work your way to more advanced positions. As a result, you will both explore each other's preferences, likes and dislikes, as well as know your limits.

Apart from the bed, another great place to start would be the living room. If you are sitting on an armchair, get her to straddle you. Her legs will be on either side of your hips and you can control her weight, getting her to put her arms around you.

In this case, you get to know her and you come extremely close. Plus, this position helps both of you to feel intense pleasure due to deep penetration. So if she is adventurous enough, do not let that opportunity pass you by. Alternatively, you can get her to lay on the sofa and work your magic.

The floor is one more fantasy coming to life, when it comes to sites for first-time sex. As long as you are feeling it, why not? At least, you can start making out on the floor then move on to the bed for a higher level of comfort. A modified 69 is great on the floor, as well as doggy style with all its variations. If you enjoy these sex positions, then you should give them a try. Obviously, you will need to check if the floor is clean enough and maybe get some pillows and a blanket to make things more comfortable. Your urge might be so intense that you literally cannot get enough of each other. If this is the case, then there is no right or wrong when choosing where to have sex for the first time. You can do it in the car or on the kitchen countertop, in the shower or even outdoors for an additional sense of adventure. Nevertheless, when you are having sex with a new partner for the first time, it is preferable to experiment and get to know them well step by step. You will have all the time in the world to try out eccentric sex positions and places that you have never even been to for love making. Set the right foundations and this is just the beginning!

Women's Little Secrets

It is not a secret that women want to be desired. And let's face it, men do too! But when it comes to women, they are particularly fond of foreplay. This is a prelude to what is coming and allows them to feel everything more intensely. It is like a decadent appetizer or amuse bouche, introducing you to the culinary wonders you are about to experience. If you truly want to stand out among the rest and become a true legend in sex, then you need to perfect your skills in foreplay. Pay attention to the signals she is sending you, take the lead and show her what you can do to make her night extra special.

Satisfying foreplay is not rushed. On the contrary, you must devote time and energy to satisfy your lady. It is so worth the time invested. Even if you do not have adequate experience, you can still do it while you get to know her better. As a result, your performance will be skyrocketing as well. Keeping that in mind, start kissing her slowly while your hands explore the curves of her body. She will be amazed at your smoothness, since you take your time and enjoy each and every inch of her skin. You will clearly realize when her heart begins beating faster and faster by the second. Whisper compliments in her ear and let her know how much you want her. Do not be afraid to express yourself, saying that she is super hot and that you would love to take her over and over again, giving her pleasure and multiple orgasms. Stimulating women does not only have to do with her body, but it also involves her mind. After seeing that she is in the mood for more action, get down on her. By that, I mean lie her down and get your lips to wander all the way from her ears to her neckline, her breasts, her belly and ultimately her thighs. This is your end destination, at least for now. Open her legs and really slowly touch and lick her inner thighs. Be careful not to dive right in between those thighs. Wait until she is craving more.

Then, when she is all wet and shaky, go for the next milestone and use your fingers and mouth, gently at first then more passionately. She will most likely have started moving to the beat of her pleasure, so follow her rhythm and make her reach an orgasm that she will never forget. But wait. This is not over. You have not conquered the territory, unless you do what most men do not care for. Give her more pleasure, until you feel that she wants you inside her. And this is when you make your move, showing her who is in control. Women love to surrender to the man who has made them reach an orgasm with such great devotion and care. (Vincenty, 2019)

Once you have reached this point, it is time for her to see how much you are enjoying yourself by finding your release. This will also make her feel desirable so don't hold back. Afterwards, feel free to tell her how much you enjoyed yourself and what she did to get you there. There is no downside to making her feel like a sexual goddess.

Chapter 15
Here is the End... or the Beginning

After a night of pure sexual pleasure, you must be feeling exhausted. You have both drained yourselves of energy, enjoying every minute of sex. But now that this is over, what next? What do you do?

Is it best to call it a day right after having sex or should you wait for a little while? Are you capable of discussing what has happened or is it just not important to talk it out? These are questions that might drive someone crazy, especially prior to having sex. However, you should not get too stressed over it. Really, if you have both loved what happened, then the odds are in your favor and it will most likely happen again soon.

Generally, it is not a great idea to fall asleep right after sex.

It is your first time together and so you must make sure that you have got some strength to keep your eyes open, at least for a while. Your special lady will want some cuddling, as you are lying together and enjoying these peaceful moments after the sex storm. It is important to promote that feeling of serenity, since it shows that you are in perfect balance with each other and can relax together.

Talking is always on the table, but it is preferable that you let her initiate the discussion. Maybe she has something on her mind and she wants to clarify some details that you might not even think about. Women tend to overanalyze any situation, after all. Bear that in mind and do not get panicked, if you are expected to answer a few questions or more than a few.

Watching TV can be fun, but after your first time sex you had better spend these moments doing better things than that. You can ask to smoke, if you feel like it. But again, respect her wishes, particularly if you are at her apartment. Of course, you might be thirsty or even hungry. Satisfy those needs of yours, because you never know when you will be up for a second round. The truth is that there is no set behavioral pattern to follow first-time sex. Every woman is different, just like you are different compared to other men. So check your chemistry, interpret the signals she is sending out to you and follow her lead again.

What to Say After Sex

We all seek validation, one way or another. This is why many people tend to ask their sex partner if they had a good time. Although this is not automatically something to avoid, you need to be subtle when asking her about her experience and level of satisfaction. "How are you feeling?" is a much better question than "Was I any good? You get the gist. Do not let your insecurities show, even if you want her to confirm that she enjoyed herself. Besides, you already know that. There is no point in pretending that she has had an orgasm, since it is your first date. If she did not get any pleasure out of the whole experience, then it is best to part ways before things get serious. Honesty is the key. Be careful not to fall for the trap of sharing emotions that you think you are feeling. Women get to express themselves more dramatically, so it should not come as a surprise if she tells you something about her feelings that you would have never said. Do not share her enthusiasm. Why say "I think I am falling for you," even if there is the slightest possibility that you are? It is way too soon to focus on anything other than physical attraction and the satisfaction you are both hopefully getting out of having sex. Some people even say "I love you" right after having sex, even though clearly they are not feeling that level of attachment yet.

Another thing that you should avoid like the plague is talking about former relationships. Why would you ever want to ruin something good, by asking those questions? There is literally no reason whatsoever why you want to know the exact number of her former lovers. These are questions that make any woman feel awkward. Unless she explicitly asks you about something similar, do not stress yourself over it. Move on. Her ex is an ex for a reason and you do not want to go down that road. Either she feels the pressure that you want to replace him or she sees that as an opportunity to compare the two of you. Neither option works in your favor.

It is needless to say that you should never ask a woman how she learned a specific thing that she did during sex. This sounds judgmental, even if your intentions are not like that. If she did something that impressed you, then you should be grateful and hope that she does that again, preferably sooner than later. In case you are wondering how come she knows these things, then you should get a grip and think of it differently. You both have a history and since she has not played the "virgin card," you cannot ask her that question. Even if she doesn't look upset or offended by that, next time (if any) she will think twice prior to using her imagination and going wild in bed.

Safe things to talk about include small talk about your professional and personal background, your hobbies and habits, your plans and dreams. "What are you doing next weekend? I would love to hang out, if you want" or "What exactly do you do at work? It must be exciting working there" or even "Is there any dream that you are hoping to achieve by the end of the year?" can be excellent topics to discuss after sex and before your next round, obviously! You can share a glass of water or a soda, grab a bite to eat or order a pizza. You can also take a shower together and leave talking for later.

What About The Next Day?

Congratulations on hitting the target, man! You have enjoyed steaming hot sex with a woman that you like and now you are wondering what to do for the next 24 hours. First of all, relax and take in what has just happened. Reminisce over those moments and think of all the good stuff that you are proud of. You must have done something right! This is your moment to shine, since you have worked hard to get where you are now. It has been a rocky path, but you have managed to cope with the challenge, lived up to expectations or even surpassed them. With the help of this book and the step-by-step guidelines that have been outlined for you, success was not in question.

Next, you have two options. Either you want to continue on with this woman or you can call it quits and move forward. If it is the former, it doesn't really matter what you do. You just let her know, before things get ugly and awkward for both of you. You can text her (which I would not recommend), call her or tell her face to face as you end this. Thank her for the moments that you spent together and just inform her that it would be best to stop right there. Be honest, but without making her feel uncomfortable or offended. You are both consenting adults, after all. It has been a pleasure and now you can part ways. This happens more often than not, as I am guessing you know by now.

If it is the latter, though, she has rocked your world and you have had great fun together. Sex has been a blast and you are surely looking forward to contacting her the next day. In fact, you must have played out all the scenarios in your mind and it feels overwhelming! Is she feeling the same? Does she want you to call so soon or is she in the need of a timeout? First things first. Take a deep breath and let's see if she shares your vibe.

A great way to follow up after a hot first time sex is to call her casually, just to see how she is doing. If she responds right away, it is clearly a sign that she has been expecting your call. But keep in mind that we all get stuck in a ton of obligations that prevent us from being available 24/7. So even if she doesn't answer your call, do not despair and wait for her to reciprocate.

Alternatively, you can text her and then wait for her reply in writing. Besides, "Verba volant, scripta manent (Spoken words fly away, written words remain) (Lymepoet, 2018). I would not recommend stopping by her office or her house, because this would seem very creepy. Give her some space and see if she sends you a message or calls you on her own. This can be fun, too. But either way, do not overthink that. If you want to meet again, you will make it happen and much sooner than you would expect.

In the meantime, it is time to reap the rewards of your hard work and then plan the rest of your strategy as to how to proceed.

For now, relax and take in that enchanting fragrance of success. You did this!

Conclusion

Relationships between men and women can be tricky. It doesn't matter if you are looking for the love of your life or a one-night stand. On any occasion, you have to make sure that you follow the steps that I have outlined in this book. Do not reveal your true intentions and do not show fear, doubts or second-guessing of your decisions. You must cultivate a specific mentality that allows you to reach your desired goal. Sex with desirable women is one of those things and you should focus on how to get it, under your own terms. Find your prey and seduce her, by following the guidelines that I shared with you. The results will be amazing! In here, I have covered all the steps that lead to female seduction and sex. Trust me, these pieces of advice have come after long hours of studying, interpreting and sharing experiences. So they have been tested and proven to work. Obviously, you will need to adjust them properly to get into a woman's heart. However, the general idea is that you need to be open, listen to her and under-stand the signals that she is sending to you. It is an interactive game, as you are not the only player.

This will not happen overnight, for sure. If you lack self-confidence or if you do not have enough experience to read between the lines of a woman's behavior, then you ought to be patient. Study her gestures, the way she talks and the things she says. Watch her smile, laugh, frown and interpret those signs. Play with her using your eyes and facial expressions, until you see that she is inviting you over. Then, apply what I have explained here and get ready to surprise her with your thoughtful gestures and patience. Step by step, even the most solid and daunting fortress will fall. You just need to be persistent.

Do not waste your time. If she does not want to talk to you, there are many other women who will. You can never know what each person is going through, so do not immediately assume that she is not interested. However, you are on a tight deadline. You should get results in seven hours or less of dealing with a woman. If you don't, then you need to move on to your next target. Do not feel guilty about that decision. You have given her a chance to know you and she has ignored that chance. So who is to blame?

It is important that you devote the time and effort needed, in order to perfect your skills and learn how to incorporate these guidelines into your everyday life. If something is troubling you, then take a moment and think about it. Play all the scenarios in your mind and practice a dialog to confront them. When you are done, practice some more. This way, you will have the opportunity to figure out how to bounce back, even when she tells you something that you do not want to hear. Besides, it is best if you are prepared for all the alternatives. This way, nothing will come as a shock to you and in fact you will be ready to respond in a witty manner that at least earns you a sincere smile.

A Whole World Unfolds Before You

Only after truly knowing your strength, will you be able to open up your eyes and understand your full potential. It is mind blowing, actually. Realizing what you are capable of can change your life. So instead of settling for mediocre things, you should focus on what you want to do then plan out your strategy as to how to achieve those things. They can be anything, from getting that promotion at work to being heard more often when you talk. There are small details that matter and you will get to see their reflection on you, as you are transforming yourself to an irresistible sex machine.

Seduction club

A whole new world filled with opportunities is gradually revealed before your very eyes. It is right there, ready for the taking. You simply need to reach out and grab what you want. The same goes for intimate relationships and your success with women. Rather than compromising with women that you do not even find attractive, just because they might be more approachable, reach for the stars. Stop settling. It will not do you any good. Instead, concentrate on your real target. Who do you want to talk to? Who do you want to have sex with? And then see how following my footsteps will help you get you to your goal.

This book has been created with the sole purpose of sharing what I have learned the hard way. It has not always been easy for me and therefore I feel like it is my duty to prepare others. Call it male solidarity, but I believe that all men should read this advice. In a perfect world, women would come with their own manual and we would not have to figure out everything from scratch. But of course, in that case we would miss out on all the fun of seduction. It is an art form and I picture all of you as artists, waiting to create your very own masterpieces.

You cannot expect to seduce every woman in your radar. Nonetheless, you will beguiled the majority of those women that you set your mind into. And this alone is something worth celebrating. Obviously, when (or if) the time comes to settle down, these guidelines can be tucked away carefully. But do not forget that you have what it takes to conquer women when you want to. This is a skill that you will never regret mastering, for sure!

Excited to Put Theory into Practice?

I have given you all the tools that you need, in order to seduce any woman in seven hours or less. Now it rests on your shoulders how to make use of this guide to your advantage. Assess your situation, know your worth and aim for your targets. Be focused on what you are looking for and do not rest until you obtain it. There might be some mistrust or self-doubt even now, after having explained everything in detail. It makes total sense why somebody might fear that theory and practice are miles apart. But here you have acquired hands-on knowledge that can be applied to everyday life quite easily. This is no generic advice like "Be yourself" or "Go over and talk to her." On the contrary, you know exactly what to do and when to do it. If you go through the chapters of the book, you will see practical information and examples that you can relate to. There is no reason for you to hold back. Go out there and prove yourself what you are made of. Stick to the plan, comply with my suggestions and follow my lead. You will get what you want, without breaking a sweat. Think of it as learning how to ride a bike. You will fall and you will fall again. In the meantime, you will be using the training wheels and you will gradually improve your skills in riding the bike. Then, one day you will realize that you do not need these training wheels any more. You will remove one of them and then the other one, while still riding and feeling the joy of accomplishment. I bet you are excited by now to get started and I share your enthusiasm.

The world is your oyster and women are waiting to be seduced by men who know how to behave and make their nights truly memorable. They are ready to say "yes." What do you say?

References

CK. (2015, February 13). Colors Speak Volumes in Gift Giving. LifeCherish.Com. https://lifecherish.com/2015/02/13/colors-in-gift-giving/

Lovz, E. (2019, March 7). 20 Body Language Signs She's Not Into You. Emlovz. https://www.emlovz.com/body-language-signs-shes-not-into-you/

Lymepoet, L. (2018, May 7). VERBA VOLANT, SCRIPTA MANENT! Steemit. https://steemit.com/life/@lymepoet/verba-volant-scripta-manent

Van Edwards, V. (2013, June 19). Female Body Language. Science of People. https://www.scienceofpeople.com/female-body-language/

Vincenty, S. (2019, August 27). For Better Foreplay, Try This. Oprah Magazine. https://www.oprahmag.com/life/relationships-love/a28829792/foreplay-tips/

Whittaker, S. (2018, July 25). How To Attract Women Without Talking – 10 Body Language Tricks To Use. Mantelligence. https://www.mantelligence.com/body-language-that-attracts-women/